This book belongs to:

_____

_____

_____

The opinions in this book reflect the research and ideas of the author but are not intended to substitute for the services of a licensed healthcare provider. Please consult your health provider before making any changes to your exercise, diet, or medication regimen.

Special thanks to Ginger Vieira for her editing, research and tireless effort to make this book even better!

For more information, visit neilgreathouse.com

TYPE ONE DIABETES - One Day at a Time
Book ISBN-13: 9798870954974

TYPE 1 DIABETES
One Day at a Time

By Neil Greathouse

I couldn't have done this without my family. You've patiently supported me for over 10 years while I write, film, edit and post ridiculous sugar-free gummy bear videos to help people living with Type 1. Thank you for all the laughter, love and inside jokes!

I love you, GreatHomes.

Gina - nurturing, life-giving, sees what's possible
Roman - visionary, man of God, steady
Sydney - joyful, focused, full of life
Cassidy - determined, artistic, maker
Cora - probably a squirrel

Endorsements from smart people

"Neil's book is like a "welcome to diabetes" letter from a friend you can trust! You can't get this information at your doctor's office — there isn't time. Easy to read, this book teaches the critical nuts and bolts of T1D without getting too complicated. Everyone diagnosed with type 1 diabetes needs this information."

~ Ginger Vieira
Author, writer & speaker

"Neil has a remarkable talent for simplifying relatable information about Type 1 Diabetes, a highly demanding disease. His knack for storytelling and simplifying information will help you relate, understand and thrive. This book is not only going to help you, but you're gonna have fun in the process. Your pancreas thanks you!"

~ Dr. Tyler Tarver
Speaker, author

"I feel like I've known Neil Greathouse my whole life. He embodies what it means to be a Diabetes Creator: identifying a need and working to meet that need in a unique creative way. I have benefitted from his videos, advice and friendship in more ways than I can count, and I know that you will benefit from his book and accompanying resources. If you or someone you love has diabetes, you have the right book. You got this!"

~ Rob Howe
Founder, Diabetics Doing Things

Yep, even more endorsements

If your T1D diagnosis felt like the universe playing a prank on you, meeting Neil Greathouse is like discovering the cosmic punchline and joining the 'Dead Pancreas Club.' Brace yourself for over 90 days of gaining practical, real-life knowledge with Neil, your newest partner in pancreas crime. He tackles each day with Type 1 using a mix of outrageous humor, humility, and authenticity, and he generously shares it all with the community. His bonus videos will have you laughing through the tears, and Neil will be there every step - from Type One, Day One and beyond. Get ready for a blood sugar rollercoaster with a side of laughter!

~ Sarah Lucas
Co-Founder & Founding CEO, Beyond Type 1

"I have known Neil since the beginning of his journey with T1D!! Watched him battle through the ups and downs and the challenges that T1D brings every day! At one point, I saw a shift in Neil from just getting by... to taking it on, learning, and gaining understanding. If you're struggling or feel defeated, this book will help you pick up your head so you can live life to the fullest."

~ Mark Pagley
Speaker & Mentor

Table of Contents

CHAPTER 1
Welcome to the Party!

Scan this before you start reading Chapter 1.

The realization hit me that seeing a doctor two or three times a year for something I have to deal with constantly didn't seem like enough.

1 WELCOME TO THE PARTY!

Let me set the scene for you! It's 1992, and I'm a 19-year-old who just spent 4 years of Air Force JROTC getting ready for this moment. I've been through 7 months of rigorous flight training, and survival training, and learned how to eat bugs or survive behind enemy lines if our plane was shot down. Every day, we trained our bodies to survive if our plane lost cabin pressure. Test after test and rigorous training was exhausting and tiring, and I freaking loved it!

I'd dreamed about this moment since I was 12 years old and started writing letters to astronauts and aviators at NASA. I begged them for any information they could give me because I'd already read every book that our local library had on the shelves. The walls of my bedroom were covered with pictures, printouts, and schematics of planes, rockets and propulsion systems. I was going to be a test pilot in the Air Force, and yeah sure, Neil Armstrong never replied to the letters I wrote him every week for two years! So what? The guy was busy, and I'm sure he had a good reason not to write back. I have zero beef with Neil Armstrong! Because I was going to be a test pilot in the United States Air Force. Except for the fact that I was very sick.

I hadn't told my roommates or fellow trainees in the Air Force that I was sick. I knew something was wrong, and I was terrified to say anything to anyone for fear of losing my flight status. I was losing weight. A lot of it. In 12 weeks, I was down about 30 pounds and had a weird, unquenchable thirst. Couldn't get enough water and had to pee almost every 30 minutes like clockwork. Something was wrong and I kept telling myself it was just stress and that I needed to push through. My vision started to get a little blurry, and I was puking at least three nights a week. The cramping in my legs kept me up at night, and the pain was unbearable.

Walking home from a training session with my best friends in our flight, I stopped along the side of the road and crumpled in a heap on the curb. I asked them to call an ambulance because I couldn't keep walking. I didn't know it yet, but my dreams of a career as a test pilot in the Air Force just ended. The hospital diagnosed me immediately with type 1 diabetes (T1D) that night, and I didn't have a clue what that meant.

Five days after I was diagnosed with T1D, the Flight Commander slowly walked into my hospital room, and I immediately felt a combination of fear and dread. I'd been in the hospital for an entire week because I had gone into diabetic ketoacidosis (DKA), and diabetes had completely shut me down. My eyesight was blurry (one of the classic symptoms of T1D) that week, but I recognized the Flight Commander's voice.

"Your flying career in the Air Force is over son," he said.

Later that week I went to my first endocrinology appointment. More information hit me than I could possibly retain. I walked out of the doctor's office with a sliding scale of how much insulin to take for my blood sugar levels scribbled out on a piece of lined notebook paper. It's not unlike when you have your first child in he hospital, and the doctors send you and your wife out to the car to take your brand-spanking new baby home.

"I have no idea what I'm doing!" I realized.

That's how I felt with T1D. What in the world am I supposed to do with all this? I don't know anyone who has it, my friends joked around with me and asked if it was catchy, and inside...my emotions were boiling.

I'd never seen a pancreas on the Operation game where you try to put the wishbone back in without touching the edges! Like, how could my pancreas do this to me when I didn't even know what it was?! So I went back home, and went to college for computer technology and creative writing — basically the exact opposite of an aviation career in the United States Air Force.

And then, on a whim, instead of taking a Certified Network Administrator test, I asked the Veterans Affairs rep to buy me a computer to edit videos. At first, they were 100% against it, and I couldn't blame them. But I kept asking, and eventually, they agreed, and I immediately started shooting videos and writing scripts and screenplays with my friends. Suddenly, I was making films. I don't know if we would have called them films back then because that sounds ultra-pretentious, but you know what I mean.

That's where I started the journey to this page you're reading now. I made YouTube videos, short films, educational videos, feature-length documentaries and everything in between. In the years since that first editing computer, we have sent 10 cameras to space and back, filmed on six continents, crashed more drones than I can count, built amazing friendships with people way more talented than me, and sat next to Oscar-winning actors in rooms where I felt like I didn't belong.

12

Through it all, I'd do my best to go to the endocrinologist a few times a year and get updates on my A1C. The realization hit me that seeing a doctor two or three times a year for something I have to deal with constantly didn't seem like enough. It couldn't be enough, right? That's a problem! That's like driving somewhere you've never been and only checking the map twice for a journey that takes a year! What if I could make helpful videos every day that broke diabetes down into smaller, bite-sized pieces that didn't overwhelm anyone? Would anybody care?

After writing, filming, and editing over 400 educational T1D videos last year, I realized that you did care! It was overwhelming to meet so many people on this T1D journey. I felt like I'd found "my people." This book is 90 days of walking alongside you as we navigate this crazy, high-maintenance disease together.

I'm not an endocrinologist, a doctor, a nurse or a brain surgeon. But what I'd like to be for you is a friend along the way between now and your next endocrinologist appointment.

Each chapter of this book covers a different topic related to the daily work and experience of living with T1D. You'll also find encouragement, challenges, and a spot to write your thoughts down.

If you'll walk through this with me, and put some of these things into practice, I believe you'll be stronger, more equipped, and more confident in your life with T1D.

CHAPTER 2
What is Type 1 Diabetes?

Scan this before you start reading Chapter 2.

The most important thing you need to know today is this: it's not your fault. You didn't do anything wrong. You didn't cause this.

WHAT IS TYPE 1 DIABETES?

This week, let's tackle the question on everyone's mind — what exactly is T1D? Simply put, it's an autoimmune disease that prevents our body from producing insulin. Unfortunately, this means that our body is essentially fighting against itself. In the case of T1D, our immune system attacks part of the pancreas that produces insulin.

T1D means our body doesn't make insulin anymore and now we need to inject it into our body. The most important thing you need to know today is this: it's not your fault. You didn't do anything wrong. You didn't cause this. (But actually, if your children or family members haven't been diagnosed, they can be screened for the earliest stages of T1D — potentially years before symptoms start! If they test positive, there are therapies that could help delay T1D. Ask your child's primary care doctor to screen them for T1D autoantibodies.)

It's something in our genetics and DNA. It's not your fault. It's not your parent's fault. It's not Little Debbie's fault. Save yourself the time and energy of trying to find out where to point the blame because it simply can't be done.

Don't think you did anything wrong — because you didn't.

Reflection:
Nobody remembers "easy".

What you're doing in managing T1D is memorable and noteworthy! It takes a lot of hard work. What is one thing that you can learn from today?

_____

_____

_____

_____

_____

_____

_____

_____

_____

_____

_____

_____

_____

_____

WHAT CAUSES TYPE 1 DIABETES?

There are these cells in the pancreas — called beta cells. Beta cells make insulin, and unfortunately, they're the ones getting targeted, attacked and destroyed by your immune system.

Over time, they make less and less insulin. We can go from "Hey, I make my own insulin" to "I'm not making any insulin" overnight or over the course of many years.. It's different for everybody.

What causes T1D is different than what triggers the full onset of the disease.

You actually started developing T1D potentially years before your blood sugar levels started rising or had any noticeable symptoms. But we know from research that you likely had autoantibodies (the result of your immune system attacking you) present in your bloodstream before you were 5 years old — even if you weren't diagnosed until many, many years later.

The trigger is what drives that quiet immune system attack into overdrive, which quickly destroys your ability to produce enough insulin, causes blood sugar levels to rise dangerously high, and results in those symptoms we all know too well.

It's often some type of stress that triggers the full onset of T1D. It could be a fever, the flu, or strep throat. Physical trauma like a car accident or breaking a bone. Stressful moments like divorce in the family or losing a loved one. Even a beneficial standard vaccine can trigger the full onset — but again, that doesn't mean it caused your T1D. Your T1D was gonna happen no matter what.

Remember, you didn't do anything to cause this. Be free of that and don't try to carry the weight of it!

Reflection:
Every day is day one.

The door is shut on yesterday, and you've got a brand new day ahead of you! What is one area that you've grown most in?

_____

_____

_____

_____

_____

_____

_____

_____

_____

_____

_____

_____

_____

_____

WHO DOES TYPE 1 DIABETES AFFECT?

Anybody can get T1D at any age. They used to call it "juvenile diabetes" because experts thought it only affected children. And that's definitely not true anymore.

Side note: I've had some people say, "You got the sugar diabetes"?! And while that's incorrect, it's also super weird! (I'm looking at you, Aunt Rita, it's not called "the sugars.")

T1D shows up at two reoccurring ages in kids, most commonly between four and seven years old and then again between 10 and 14 years old.

About 250,000 kids in America have T1D, compared to the 1.5 million adults who have it. I have good friends who were diagnosed in their 30s, 40s and 50s! It's actually just as common in adults as children today.

The full onset in adults often takes longer, which makes it harder for doctors to diagnose it accurately. T1D in adults is often misdiagnosed as type 2 diabetes (T2D) simply because many doctors still think it only develops in childhood.

T1D also affects males and females almost equally. Two days ago, I got another call from a family friend whose son was diagnosed with T1D after his football practice, and it blindsided them! Diabetes doesn't have a lot of respect for who it affects.

Reflection:
You're not doing a bad job; you're doing a difficult job.

Numbers are just numbers — not "good or bad." What is something you can celebrate that you did well today?

_____

_____

_____

_____

_____

_____

_____

_____

_____

_____

_____

_____

_____

_____

WHAT ARE THE ODDS OF GETTING TYPE 1 DIABETES?

Get this: 85 to 90 percent of all T1D cases are in people with no family history of the disease! That's another reason why everybody should be screening their children for the autoantibodies of T1D before symptoms start.

As far as I know, no one in my family has ever had T1D. So when the doctors told me I had it, I was kind of shocked.

Having a "first—degree family member" (a parent or a sibling) with T1D increases our odds of being diagnosed.

- The risk of developing T1D with no family history — 0.4%
- If our biological mother has T1D — the risk is 1 — 4 %
- If our biological father has T1D — the risk is 3 — 8%
- And if both our biological parents have T1D — the risk is as high as 30%

Scientists won't say that it's entirely genetic. All they'll agree on is "there's a strong genetic component" to T1D.

Reflection:

We are building resilience in us! We're stronger for it and more capable than we ever knew!

Resilience is our superpower, living with T1D. It's building muscles in us that we would never think to work out! What is one thing you can do for yourself today?

_____

_____

_____

_____

_____

_____

_____

_____

_____

_____

_____

_____

_____

_____

TYPE 1 AND TYPE 2 DIABETES

A lot of times, people use the word "diabetes," and they don't realize that T1D and T2D are very different. One isn't better than the other — this isn't a diabetes contest!

T1D is autoimmune and we don't make any insulin. T2D is a progressive metabolic disease where the body has become resistant to insulin and can gradually struggle to produce normal amounts of insulin over time.

Most of the time, people living with T2D treat it through lifestyle changes, oral medications, or insulin. About 10–20% of people living with T2D also take insulin to make up for the deficiency of their body needs. While it's believed that T2D can simply be cured by exercising and losing weight, this isn't true. Research on T2D shows that it's highly related to your genetics, and many people with T2D will need medications and/or insulin despite healthy lifestyle choices.

Currently, about 1.3 million people live with T1D in the US, and nearly 30 million people live with T2D in the US. On average, one out of every 10 adults over 20 years old has T2D. No matter what type of diabetes a person is living with, we're all in this together!

Reflection:
What we celebrate grows.

The things we fist pump and applaud are the things that flourish.
Who has been your biggest support this week?

_____

_____

_____

_____

_____

_____

_____

_____

_____

_____

_____

_____

_____

_____

DIFFERENT TYPES OF DIABETES

How many different types of diabetes are there? If you guessed 10 — BINGO! Please sit by your front door and wait for the mailman to bring you your prize! (it's one of those giant stuffed elephants you see at the county fair but can never actually win) The most common types of Diabetes are T1D, T2D, gestational diabetes, and Latent Autoimmune Diabetes in Adults (LADA).

Gestational diabetes can develop during pregnancy in women who previously haven't been affected by diabetes. Women will have higher blood sugar and need to take extra care of themselves and their baby. This one usually goes away after giving birth to their tiny tot!

LADA sits right between T2D and T1D, all sneaky—like. Some symptoms are like T1D, and others act like T2D, which is why it's commonly referred to as Type 1.5. Typically, this happens to adults and takes months to progress, making a diagnosis much trickier. It can be described as an "extremely slow-developing" form of T1D.

Reflection:
The highs and lows will happen, but it's what we do with the in-between moments that count!

Away from the anxious moments, the math, the medicine...what did you learn that will benefit you next week and next month?

_____

_____

_____

_____

_____

_____

_____

_____

_____

_____

_____

_____

_____

_____

HOW DO I GET DIAGNOSED WITH TYPE 1 DIABETES?

We can "find out" we have T1D in a few different ways.

The first way is to check your blood sugar. You prick your finger and put a drop of blood in a glucometer, it will tell us what your blood sugar number is. If it's high, or very high, that means your body needs insulin.

The second is an A1C test. This is a short name for "glycosylated hemoglobin test." (That sounds like a villain in a Marvel movie.) It measures your average blood sugar levels over 3 months by checking how much glucose (the sugar in your blood) is sticking to your red blood cells.

The third way is to check for autoantibodies. This is a byproduct of your immune system when it mistakenly attacks your pancreas. If there are autoantibodies, it's almost a guarantee that you've got T1D (or LADA) because these don't show up in someone with type 2. (If you've been diagnosed with T2D and an autoantibody test comes back positive, it means you've been diagnosed with the wrong type of diabetes!)

Reflection:
Good habits must be established before they can be improved.

You're out there doing the hard work of balancing T1D and life!
What is one thing that's working well for you?

CHAPTER 3

All about insulin

Scan this before you start reading Chapter 3.

Back in 1921, a Canadian scientist named Frederick Banting and his assistant Charles Best "discovered insulin."

WHAT IS INSULIN?

Insulin is a hormone produced by your pancreas. and it helps your body turn glucose into energy. It moves sugar from your blood into cells all over your body. It's like a key that opens the doors to the cells in your body.

When that door is open, the glucose in your blood can move to the cells that need it in your muscles, your brain, your eyes, your kidneys, and even your biceps. I don't recommend injecting insulin directly into the bicep for a lot of reasons, especially if "swole is your goal." (I apologize for that one.)

If you're not successfully making your own insulin, in the case of T1D — you'll need to take insulin daily with injections, a pump, or inhalation. For me, I've been doing this for 11,499 days. Not a single day off. Proud of you guys out there doing this every day. You're stronger for it — more resilient for it, better equipped to handle anything life throws at us. (And actually, you're still alive because you're still doing it!)

Reflection:
The old you isn't the new you.

Today is brand new, and so are you! You're wiser for having gone through yesterday and learned something. Name one area that you've grown the most.

_____

_____

_____

_____

_____

_____

_____

_____

_____

_____

_____

_____

_____

WHAT IS THE HISTORY OF INSULIN?

Back in 1921, a Canadian scientist named Frederick Banting and his assistant Charles Best "discovered insulin." Basically, they removed insulin from a dog's pancreas and then helped save other dogs and animals with diabetes.

Then they helped humans who had diabetes! On January 11, 1922, Leonard Thompson, a 14-year-old with T1D, became the first person to receive an insulin injection to treat T1D. His first injection: he had an allergic reaction to it, and they refined it. Twelve days later, on January 23rd, his second injection was more successful.

Before that injection, Leonard was gradually starving to death while his blood glucose and ketone levels were rising to life-threatening levels. His life would've been cut very, very short.

Dr. Banting won the Nobel Prize in medicine because until then, people with T1D only had one way of "treating" it — starvation diets. That is, they extended their lives slightly by not eating. Which you and I know isn't effective or a cure; it was a death sentence.

Reflection:
Be honest with yourself about how you're feeling today.

Take a minute and breathe in how you feel, without judgment. What can you be honest about that maybe you've been tiptoeing around before?

_____

_____

_____

_____

_____

_____

_____

_____

_____

_____

_____

_____

_____

_____

_____

WHAT ARE THE TYPES OF INJECTIBLE INSULIN?

There are SO MANY different types of insulins that pharmaceutical companies have developed over the years — including rapid-acting, long-acting, and everything in between.

On average, rapid-acting insulins take effect between 15—30 minutes and last for 3+ hours. They have been engineered to peak around 1—2 hours after injection where they're most effective, and slowly fall off afterward. These are usually taken in conjunction with meals or to correct a high blood sugar.

The other primary type of insulin is called long-acting. Catchy, I know. These are taken once or twice a day and are considered "basal insulins" (more on that in the next few chapters). They last for 24 hours and are like a slow drip that doesn't have a huge spike of effectiveness but more like a constant effect. Think of this as the classic case of the tortoise and the hare.

INSULIN	ONSET	PEAK	DURATION
Fiasp (aspart)	2 to 15 minutes	30 to 60 minutes	4 hours
Novolog (aspart)	15 minutes	45 minutes	3 to 5 hours
Humalog (lispro)	15 minutes	45 minutes	3 to 5 hours
Apidra (glulisine)	15 minutes	60 minutes	2 to 4 hours
Afrezza (inhaled)	4 to 15 minutes	35 to 45 minutes	1.5 to 3 hours

Reflection:
Nobody remembers "easy".

What you're doing in managing T1D is memorable and noteworthy!
It takes a lot of hard work. What is one thing that you can learn
from today?

_____

_____

_____

_____

_____

_____

_____

_____

_____

_____

_____

_____

_____

TAKING INSULIN VIA INJECTION OR INSULIN PUMP

It may be obvious, but there are many different ways you can make this happen. Insulin used to come in vials where you'd take a syringe, fill it up with the amount you need, and inject it into a fatty portion of your body like the abdomen, hips, thighs, buttocks or back of the arm. (I snickered typing the word "buttocks.")

Insulin pens take that concept and combine it where we simply swap out the pen needle and keep the insulin in a tiny pen that dials up the exact dosage. Both syringes and insulin pens are considered MDI — multiple daily injections — and the majority of people across the globe use this method to take insulin.

If you're one of the ones using an insulin pump, congratulations! These have a tiny tube (a cannula) that's inserted under the skin for about 3 days. The insulin pump is programmed with estimates of your body's insulin needs, and where provides a constant drip as a basal rate. For meals and corrections, it can give larger doses. or different doses of insulin.

There are trade-offs to insulin pumps vs. injections, but most people find pumps are easier because they do a lot more of the mental T1D work for you. Today's pumps also include "closed-loop" pumps that do even more of the thinking for you!

Reflection:
Every day is day one.

The door is shut on yesterday, and you've got a brand new day ahead of you! What is one area that you've grown most in?

_____

_____

_____

_____

_____

_____

_____

_____

_____

_____

_____

_____

_____

_____

_____

HOW DOES INHALED INSULIN WORK?

Most of us inject insulin through a pump, syringe, or insulin pen, but there's another method out there! Inhaled insulin is in the "ultra rapid-acting" category, and people with T1D and T2D can take it. Keep in mind though, that you can't just swap out the insulin you inject and inhale the same amount. It requires a bit of learning and patience because the dosing and how it works in your body is quite different.

Inhaled insulin passes through the lining of your lungs, where it enters the bloodstream. This is considered "pulmonary delivery," and it's very fast. Much faster than an injection — but that comes with some drawbacks. While it's the fastest on the market to enter your bloodstream, it doesn't last as long in your bloodstream, either.

Inhaled insulin can be used to cover the insulin for your meals and correcting high blood sugar levels.

This can't replace your long-acting or basal insulin. You'll also still need to take a basal/background insulin via injection (long-acting) or pump (basal rate) along with inhaled insulin.

Reflection:

You're not doing a bad job; you're doing a difficult job.

Numbers are just numbers — not "good or bad." What is something you can celebrate that you did well today?

_____

_____

_____

_____

_____

_____

_____

_____

_____

_____

_____

_____

_____

_____

DOES GENERIC INSULIN EXIST?

We haven't really talked about how expensive insulin is. (I did a series of videos on this if you want to watch, but it gets kinda dicey). Would a generic insulin or a cheaper version of insulin be a good thing?

The earliest forms of insulin were made from cow and pig insulin until 1978. But that caused quite a few problems with allergic reactions.

That's when the first "synthetic human insulin" was made. Then in 1982 came the first biosynthetic human insulin called Humulin. The most prominent insulin manufacturers are Eli Lilly, Novo Nordisk and Sanofi, but companies like CivicaRX.

They will produce something called "biosimilars," which will be cheaper. Anytime you see biosimilar insulin or other drugs — it's typically 15% to 35% lower than the name-brand version.

Reflection:

We are building resilience in us! We're stronger for it and more capable than we ever knew!

Resilience is our superpower, living with T1D. It's building muscles in us that we would never think to work out! What is one thing you can do for yourself today?

_____

_____

_____

_____

_____

_____

_____

_____

_____

_____

_____

_____

_____

_____

HOW DO YOU STORE INSULIN?

Insulin is a pretty fragile hormone and should be stored in a refrigerator at home. Ideally, put it on a center shelf. This way, it doesn't freeze in the back of the fridge where nobody ever sees it. If you haven't opened or used the insulin bottle, you can keep it at room temperature for 28 days, but after those 28 days, it won't be as effective. Insulin can survive unopened for well over a year (look at the expiration date on the box!). But once you open it and start using it, insulin generally starts to degrade after about 28 days. It simply becomes less effective.

There will be two dates on any insulin bottle — one says "use by," and one says "expiration" date. You may want to write down the date you opened the insulin bottle.

If your insulin is exposed to temperatures above 98.6 degrees Fahrenheit — pitch it. It's no good. And if it's ever frozen or in temperatures below -4 degrees Fahrenheit, pitch it. Insulin that's frozen can't hurt us — it just won't work. It's no good.

In general, don't leave your insulin in a hot car or sitting in the sun on a beach. Don't leave it in a freezing cold car, sitting in a snow bank, or exposed to New England temperatures in February while you're skating on your neighbor's pond. Keep your insulin safe from extreme temperatures.

Reflection:
What we celebrate grows.

The things we fist pump and applaud are the things that flourish.
Who has been your biggest support this week?

_____

_____

_____

_____

_____

_____

_____

_____

_____

_____

_____

_____

_____

_____

CHAPTER 4

Blood Sugar

Scan this before you start reading Chapter 4.

It's important to remember these are just numbers. The numbers themselves aren't bad or good — they have no feelings.

WHAT IS BLOOD GLUCOSE?

Blood glucose is a number or "level" representing how much sugar is in your bloodstream. It's not really sugar, like simple table sugar — but some people call it "blood sugar." It's really blood glucose.

There are so many things that can affect your blood glucose levels. The most common is what you eat or drink. Other things include stress, altitude, exercise, caffeine, hormones, medications (like steroids), or if we're sick with a cold or fever. And here's the shocking one: your own body can produce and store glucose. Without even asking, your body can release that stored glucose, spiking your blood glucose like whoa. Actually, even exercise can convert lactic acid into glucose! Evil wizardry? Sabotage!

In T1D, your blood glucose values can feel wildly out of your control, fluctuating all over the place even when you're following your doctor's directions! The reality is: managing blood glucose levels is really complicated because you're juggling so many factors, many of which you can't predict or control. That's not ideal, and we want our blood glucose levels to be between 70 and 99 mg/dL without any food in our digestive system. That's considered the "normal range" in people without diabetes.

Reflection:
The highs and lows will happen, but it's what we do with the in-between moments that count!

Away from the anxious moments, the math, the medicine...what did you learn that will benefit you next week and next month?

_____

_____

_____

_____

_____

_____

_____

_____

_____

_____

_____

_____

_____

_____

WHY SHOULD YOU CHECK YOUR BG?

Checking blood glucose levels is super important, and there are a couple of ways to do this, but the most common is with a glucometer. Most people call this their "meter".

Checking your blood glucose tells you how much insulin you need or if you need to eat or drink something with carbohydrates. You'll get a blood glucose level on a glucometer or continuous glucose monitor (CGM), which gives you the information you need to make careful decisions around food or insulin. If the numbers are consistently out of your goal range, that likely means it's time to talk to your healthcare team and make some adjustments to your medications.

It's important to remember these are just numbers. The numbers themselves aren't bad or good — they have no feelings. And you shouldn't blame yourself or beat yourself up when you see a number outside of the ideal range.

A1C	Average BG	Range of BG
5%	97 mg/dL	76-120 range
6%	126 mg/dL	100-152 range
7%	154 mg/dL	123-185 range
8%	183 mg/dL	147-217 range
9%	212 mg/dL	170-249 range
10%	240 mg/dL	193-282 range
11%	269 mg/dL	217-314 range
12%	298 mg/dL	240-347 range

Reflection:

Good habits must be established before they can be improved.

You're out there doing the hard work of balancing T1D and life! What is one thing that's working well for you?

_____

_____

_____

_____

_____

_____

_____

_____

_____

_____

_____

_____

_____

_____

WHAT ARE GLUCOMETERS?

There are around 140 different kinds of blood glucose meters on the market. Pick one that works best for you. Some connect to your phone, some to an insulin pump. Just pick the one that works best for you! (You can also get glucometers and strips from online companies like OneDrop and Diathrive without insurance limitations.)

Along with your glucometer, a few other things come in the container. Lancets help prick your fingers so you can put a tiny drop of blood on the tip of the test strip. These test strips have chemicals on them that interact with your blood, and the meter can run a tiny electrical current through the test strip to give us a blood glucose reading.

Most glucometers give a result in about 5 seconds, and some even connect to your smartphone or computer. They even have internal memory that can store the results for a long time. How long? Maaaaaaaaan, a long time. (I don't know because they're all different.)

Reflection:
The old you isn't the new you.

Today is brand new, and so are you! You're wiser for having gone through yesterday and learned something. Name one area that you've grown the most.

WHAT IS AN A1C TEST?

The number on your glucometer is just one snapshot of your blood glucose. It's constantly changing, and it's like taking a family photo that we can look at, and everybody loves, but there were thousands of other pictures before & after that moment. Screaming kids, people with their eyes closed, the dog not cooperating, or Aunt Rita with lipstick on her teeth. Those are all the things we don't see. The same thing happens with your blood.

A hemoglobin A1C test is called "A1C" for short, and it's a 2-3 month average of your blood glucose levels. You'll typically get an A1C done at your doctor's office.

A1C basically measures how much glucose is stuck to your red blood cells. And your A1C result actually translates to an average blood glucose level, so it gives you a good idea of where your BG is generally hanging out most of the time.

The goal for most adults with T1D is an A1C below 7%. That translates to a blood glucose level of around 154 mg/dL.

Reflection:
Be honest with yourself about how you're feeling today.

Take a minute and breathe in how you feel, without judgment. What can you be honest about that maybe you've been tiptoeing around before?

_____

_____

_____

_____

_____

_____

_____

_____

_____

_____

_____

_____

_____

_____

WHAT IS A CGM?

The first continuous glucose monitor (CGM) was approved by the FDA back in 1999. I wore one of these back in 2004. It was bulky and weird looking. This device measures the amount of glucose in the "interstitial fluid" in the tissue that's just under the skin — this same tissue where you inject insulin. It's not measuring your blood glucose, but the number is eventually the same as the glucose in your blood. The glucose in that interstitial fluid eventually moves its way into your bloodstream.

Thanks to CGM technology, we now have time-in-range (TIR) to help us analyze our glucose levels and overall diabetes management. TIR is the percentage of time that a person spends with their blood glucose levels in a target range. (More on this in a bit!)

Reflection:
Nobody remembers "easy".

What you're doing in managing T1D is memorable and noteworthy! It takes a lot of hard work. What is one thing that you can learn from today?

_____

_____

_____

_____

_____

_____

_____

_____

_____

_____

_____

_____

_____

WHAT IS TIME-IN-RANGE?

If you legit want to show T1D who's boss, you know, do some trash-talking to T1D, TIR is the way to go. It gives you a much more detailed idea of your blood glucose levels than an A1C test.

The goals that are recommended for TIR are:
- In range: At least 70% of the day — between 70-180 mg/dL.
- Above range: Less than 25% of the day above 180 mg/dL
- Below range: Less than 4% of the day above 250 mg/dL
- Very below range: And less than 4% of the day below 70 mg/dL

TIR is so important because it helps you start recognizing patterns. If you're realizing, "Oh wow, I'm typically high in the morning when I wake up," or "My blood glucose seems to be lower at night after dinner," then you can make adjustments.

It also helps you and your doctor spot if you're spending a lot of time low (below range) or a lot of time high (above range). While A1C just paints a vague picture of your blood glucose levels, TIR reveals more about your daily quality of life and safety with T1D.

Getting TIR data means using a continuous glucose monitor (CGM) because it's pretty darn hard to get all that data with fingersticks. TIR data is probably the most valuable data you can get to help you manage life with diabetes.

Let's say that your doctor was actually Nicholas Cage in the new National Treasure 3 movie, and he's running all over the globe; he'd be trying to get ahold of your TIR data. Plus, he'd look cool doing it. That one makes no sense, sorry.

Reflection:
Every day is day one.

The door is shut on yesterday, and you've got a brand new day ahead of you! What is one area that you've grown most in?

_____

_____

_____

_____

_____

_____

_____

_____

_____

_____

_____

_____

_____

_____

IS TIR MORE ACCURATE THAN A1C?

TIR is a way for us to measure the highs, lows and in-range values throughout the day. TIR is more informative because an A1C only gives us an average over a few months. It can't show us how much time we spend with high, low, or in-range blood glucose levels during the day.

An A1C is like trying to summarize an entire 3-month summer break away in one photo. That photo can't possibly reflect the highs and low moments that happened over three months. It is possible to have lots of high and low blood sugar readings in those three months but have an average that appears to be in range. TIR also has the added benefit of standard deviation (SD). SD is a way of measuring the range of blood glucose readings around our average. If you have had many highs or lows throughout the day, your SD will be a larger number. In contrast, if your blood sugars have been fairly stable, the SD will be a lower number.

For the most part, clinicians recommend seeing an SD be less than ⅓ of our average blood glucose. This gives our doctors a good indication if we are having significant rises or falls in our blood sugars and not just our average blood sugar. This is why TIR is a much clearer picture of our blood sugar than an A1C!

Reflection:
You're not doing a bad job; you're doing a difficult job.

Numbers are just numbers — not "good or bad." What is something you can celebrate that you did well today?

_____

_____

_____

_____

_____

_____

_____

_____

_____

_____

_____

_____

_____

_____

CHAPTER 5

Low Blood Sugar

Scan this before you start reading Chapter 5.

The reason you feel like doo doo when your blood goes low is because your brain cannot function without glucose.

WHAT IS LOW BLOOD SUGAR?

What is actually happening in your body when your blood sugar drops low? It's dangerous, and for many of us living with T1D, it's our kryptonite. The medical term for "low blood glucose" is hypoglycemia. People in the diabetes community will most likely say, "I'm low."

What is considered low? Well, that's different for people with and without diabetes!

For those of us living with T1D, the clinical definition is when your blood sugar drops below 70 mg/dL. But for people without diabetes, it's anything below 65 mg/dL, which is a lot lower because they're at less risk of continuing to go low or getting to the "life-threatening" part.

Your brain cannot function without glucose. Every second, your brain relies on the delivery of glucose! Your body is getting glucose from the food you eat (including carbohydrates and protein) and your liver's stored glucose. The reason you feel like doo doo when your blood goes low is because your brain cannot function without glucose.

Reflection:
We are building resilience in us! We're stronger for it and more capable than we ever knew!

Resilience is our superpower, living with T1D. It's building muscles in us that we would never think to work out! What is one thing you can do for yourself today?

_____
_____
_____
_____
_____
_____
_____
_____
_____
_____
_____
_____
_____

WHAT ARE THE SYMPTOMS OF LOW BLOOD SUGAR?

The symptoms of a low could look like this for us:
- Shaking or trembling
- Fast heart rate
- Extreme hunger
- Sweating or chills
- Confusion
- Difficulty concentrating
- Dizziness
- Tingling in your lips, tongue or cheeks
- Your brain is low on battery because your blood sugar is so low.

And those are just for hypoglycemia. It gets more drastic when you get to severe hypoglycemia:
- Blurred vision or double vision
- Slurred speech
- Clumsiness or feeling like you're falling
- Seizures or loss of consciousness

The effects of hypoglycemia aren't just for the moment, either. The intense food cravings. The headache. The exhaustion. The all-around feeling like you've been run over by a dump truck can last for hours or even a whole day. Every single person with T1D has felt a low blood sugar, so you're not alone!

Reflection:
What we celebrate grows.

The things we fist pump and applaud are the things that flourish.
Who has been your biggest support this week?

_____

_____

_____

_____

_____

_____

_____

_____

_____

_____

_____

_____

_____

_____

_____

WHAT IS GLUCAGON?

What is the exact opposite of insulin? It's something called glucagon, and the pancreas produces it. A healthy pancreas produces insulin from beta cells and glucagon from alpha cells. Glucagon raises your blood sugar! Glucagon is a hormone that raises blood glucose by telling your liver to release stored glucose (glycogen) and convert it into glucose — a process known as glycogenolysis.

If you or someone close to you experiences a severe drop in blood sugar levels, administering glucagon is the next course of action. A blood glucose level below 54 mg/dL is considered dangerously low. At this point, you may feel weak and have difficulty standing or functioning independently, and there is a risk of passing out. You'd give a glucagon injection to raise your blood sugar levels, and it happens in about 15-30 minutes.

You might think you don't need glucagon if you can feel your lows — but there are a variety of reasons to keep glucagon on hand. Ever gotten a stomach virus? Imagine puking your entire dinner, can't keep food down at all, and knowing you have a big bolus of rapid-acting insulin in your system! That would be a good time to have glucagon nearby.

Don't have any glucagon? Talk to your doctor! Every person taking insulin should also get and fill a prescription for emergency glucagon. Today's single-step glucagon tools make treating severe hypoglycemia with glucagon easier than it used to be:
- Zegalogue: Auto-injection Pen or Prefilled Syringe (PFS)
- Gvoke: HypoPen or Prefilled Syringe (PFS)
- Baqsimi: (nasal spray)
- GEK: the old-school multi-step glucagon emergency kit

Reflection:

The highs and lows will happen, but it's what we do with the in-between moments that count!

Away from the anxious moments, the math, the medicine...what did you learn that will benefit you next week and next month?

_____

_____

_____

_____

_____

_____

_____

_____

_____

_____

_____

_____

_____

_____

_____

WHAT CAUSES LOW BLOOD SUGAR?

A lot of different things can cause your blood sugars to drop below 70 mg/dL, and knowing what causes them is the first step in helping to prevent them. Just understand, it's unrealistic to think you'll never have a low — they happen. Trust me, they can be sneaky.

Giving too much insulin for the food you're trying to dose for can cause us to drop low. Or waiting too long in between meals to eat while a long-acting insulin is still in your system can make us drop slowly.

Insulin isn't the only thing that can cause a low! Activities like walking, running, playing in the park or swimming can tank your blood sugars. When you have insulin on board (in your body), it works faster than if you were just sitting at home watching TV. So be aware that activity can definitely play a big part in causing a low blood sugar moment!

Reflection:
Good habits must be established before they can be improved.

You're out there doing the hard work of balancing T1D and life! What is one thing that's working well for you?

_____
_____
_____
_____
_____
_____
_____
_____
_____
_____
_____
_____
_____
_____

HOW DO YOU TREAT LOW BLOOD SUGAR?

Have you heard the old 15 - 15 rule? It's old advice that if you experience a low, to eat 15 grams of carbohydrates, then wait 15 minutes and recheck your blood sugar. But the 15:15 rule doesn't work for all the different kinds of low blood sugars.

Think about it. If you're dangerously low, eating 15 grams and waiting 15 minutes may not be really smart. Sure, if it's a mild low, be careful and measure out 15 grams. If it's a severe low or a double arrow down and your CGM says you're at 50 mg/dL, don't just eat 15 grams. You'll need more rapid-acting carbohydrates — potentially 25 or 30 grams. You might need even more if you're in the middle of exercise.

Eat or drink fast-acting carbohydrates — which means starchy or sugary foods that don't contain a lot of fat or protein. Glucose tabs are the fastest because they contain a type of sugar called dextrose, which is identical to the sugar in your bloodstream.

Don't have fancy glucose tabs? A juice box or candy that doesn't have a lot of fiber, fat, or other stuff in it is a good start. Skittles, Airheads, fruit snacks, Smarties, Starburst...the list goes on! I personally use Sunkist fruit gems because they have little wrappers and are about 8 grams of carbs each.

Reflection:
The old you isn't the new you.

Today is brand new, and so are you! You're wiser for having gone through yesterday and learned something. Name one area that you've grown the most.

_____

_____

_____

_____

_____

_____

_____

_____

_____

_____

_____

_____

_____

_____

WHAT ARE THE COMPLICATIONS OF LOW BLOOD SUGAR?

Yes, severe hypoglycemia can kill you. But even mild-to-moderate lows can cause long-term damage to your brain.

This has been a topic of debate among doctors for years. Previously, it was believed that hypoglycemia starved brain cells of glucose, but recent studies say this isn't entirely accurate. Brain cells actually die when their electrical activity stops as glucose levels drop below 18 mg/dL. Aspartate is a substance released in your brain, and those brain cells can't survive.

Without enough glucose and then enough aspartate, you have a hard time thinking because you're losing some of the fuel for your brain to function. Think of it like a car running out of gas. It doesn't immediately stop running — it sputters for a bit. The more lows you have, the more likely you are to not "feel them" as much, which is dangerous.

You don't want to live on the verge of passing out or your brain losing function because it does long-term damage to your ability to reason and make healthy decisions.

Research on frequent hypoglycemia has also found it increases your risk for things like dementia. Enduring lots of lows is not a good way to live! Talk to your doctor if you're experiencing frequent hypoglycemia — most likely, it means your insulin doses need some major tweaking!

Reflection:
Be honest with yourself about how you're feeling today.

Take a minute and breathe in how you feel, without judgment.
What can you be honest about that maybe you've been tiptoeing
around before?

_____

_____

_____

_____

_____

_____

_____

_____

_____

_____

_____

_____

_____

_____

WHAT HAPPENS WHEN YOU ARE HYPOGLYCEMIC UNAWARE?

Hypo Unawareness is when your body doesn't "feel" the symptoms of low blood sugar, and it's super sneaky. Typically, those symptoms kick in when your blood sugars fall below 54 mg/dL (3.0 mmol/L). But with hypoglycemia unawareness, you might not feel the usual shakiness, hunger, or sweating – the "autonomic" symptoms. Autonomic refers to things that your body doesn't automatically. The longer you've lived with T1D, the more likely you've experienced some damage to your autonomic system, and thus, your ability to feel lows.

Other factors that can impair your ability to feel the symptoms of lows include while you're exercising or while you're asleep. Thankfully, CGMs can help keep you safer during both of these activities!

You're not alone. About 1 in 5 people with T1D say they experience hypo unawareness. And insulin-dependent T2Ds deal with it, too!

Reflection:
Nobody remembers "easy".

What you're doing in managing T1D is memorable and noteworthy! It takes a lot of hard work. What is one thing that you can learn from today?

_____

_____

_____

_____

_____

_____

_____

_____

_____

_____

_____

_____

_____

_____

CHAPTER 6

High Blood Sugar

Scan this before you start reading Chapter 6.

High blood sugars are really caused by everyday challenges in the juggling act of insulin vs. food vs. activity. Plus, a whole mess of other factors!

WHAT IS CONSIDERED HIGH BLOOD SUGAR?

High blood sugar can be damaging to our body over time, and the medical term for high BG is hyperglycemia. To be honest, I deal with my blood sugar going higher more often than I deal with it going low.

According to the ADA, anything outside the 70-180 mg/dL range is considered harmful. In a person without diabetes, anything over 140 mg/dL is generally considered high. For people with T1D, the general goal is to stay below 180 mg/dL because it's realistically achievable for many people — but still very challenging!

What happens when your blood glucose is higher is pretty fascinating. (Better to stay curious than to get fearful, right?) Elevated levels over a long period of time mean your body has a more challenging time getting oxygen to your cells, then inflammation sets in and your organs and blood vessels don't like that.

In a nutshell: high blood sugars can damage and destroy nerves and blood vessels throughout nearly every part of your body. The more often your blood sugar is high, the more damage your body is enduring. The more often your blood sugar is high, the greater your risk of developing diabetes-related complications like retinopathy (in your eyes), nephropathy (in your kidneys), neuropathy (in your fingers and toes), etc.

Reflection:
Every day is day one.

The door is shut on yesterday, and you've got a brand new day ahead of you! What is one area that you've grown most in?

_____

_____

_____

_____

_____

_____

_____

_____

_____

_____

_____

_____

_____

_____

_____

WHAT ARE THE SYMPTOMS OF HIGH BLOOD SUGAR?

High blood sugars have a few very important signs and symptoms, and it's essential for us to know what they are. Some common symptoms of persistently high blood sugar include:
- Excessive thirst
- Frequent urination
- Fatigue
- Blurred vision
- Slow-healing wounds

More sudden and immediate symptoms of high blood sugar are a little different. When your blood sugar spikes after eating or missing an insulin dose, for example, the immediate symptoms of high blood sugar include:
- Sudden irritability
- Cravings (even if you just ate)
- Sudden drowsiness
- Headache
- Thirst
- Difficulty concentrating

The higher your blood sugar is, and the longer it's high, the more severe your symptoms can become. Blood sugar levels over 250 mg/dL can increase your risk of ketones and diabetic ketoacidosis (DKA). More on DKA in a moment!

If you're experiencing frequent high blood sugars, it's definitely a sign that your insulin doses and other medications need some fine-tuning with support from your healthcare team. Don't endure the highs — reach out for help! And as thankful as we are for our body trying to keep us healthy, this leads to very dangerous results called Diabetic Ketoacidosis (DKA).

Reflection:
You're not doing a bad job; you're doing a difficult job.

Numbers are just numbers — not "good or bad." What is something you can celebrate that you did well today?

_____

_____

_____

_____

_____

_____

_____

_____

_____

_____

_____

_____

_____

_____

WHAT IS DKA? (DIABETIC KETOACIDOSIS)

A lot of people, when they're first diagnosed with T1D, go into DKA. DKA means diabetic ketoacidosis. It's the big bad wolf. DKA occurs when there is too little insulin available in your bloodstream. It can develop:

- In the weeks and months before your diagnosis
- If you forget to take your insulin
- If your insulin pump malfunctions and doesn't deliver insulin properly
- If your insulin is damaged (by extreme temperatures) and thus not potent
- If you come down with "regular people sickness" like the flu
- If you vomit excessively due to a stomach virus (severe dehydration) and more

About 46 percent of patients who get T1D, go into DKA when they're diagnosed. What happens in DKA: your body tries to rescue you when there isn't enough insulin present. If you don't have enough insulin in your system, your body starts burning fat for energy — and the byproduct of that type of fat-burning is ketones. Think of it like exhaust from a car when the engine is burning fuel.

Ketones alone aren't bad, but too much can be deadly because they're acidic. At low levels, ketones are actually common and normal — like if you skip breakfast, you probably have low levels of ketones present. But, ketone levels associated with a lack of insulin can be deadly. You can test your ketones with urine strips (from the pharmacy) or a blood ketone meter. It doesn't matter your age or how much T1D experience you have — DKA can happen to anybody. The most important thing to know about DKA: don't try to manage it at home! Call your doctor and go to the ER for intravenous fluids to help you get back on track. DKA will likely only get worse if you try to cope at home.

Reflection:
We are building resilience in us! We're stronger for it and more capable than we ever knew!

Resilience is our superpower, living with T1D. It's building muscles in us that we would never think to work out! What is one thing you can do for yourself today?

_____

_____

_____

_____

_____

_____

_____

_____

_____

_____

_____

_____

_____

_____

WHAT CAUSES HIGH BLOOD SUGAR?

High blood sugars are really caused by everyday challenges in the juggling act of insulin vs. food vs. activity. Plus, a whole mess of other factors! Here are a few things that can cause high BGs:

- Not enough rapid-acting insulin with meals
- Not enough basal/long-acting insulin (your needs can change)
- Hormones like adrenaline, cortisol, dopamine
- Caffeine (maybe not one cup, but two cups, etc. — everybody's different!)
- Menstruation
- Dehydration
- Steroids
- Stress
- Illness (flu, cold, strep, fever, etc.)
- Excitement (like roller coaster rides, job promotions, your wedding day, etc.)
- Growth hormones (growing up usually means insulin needs to go up, too!)
- ...and more!

Stress can cause our blood glucose levels to rise because of the different hormones that occur in the body, like adrenaline, cortisol or dopamine. These can raise our levels without us even being aware of it and can get sneaky. If we have the flu or another virus making us sick, our body goes into repair mode, and that can sometimes raise our levels as well. Be careful to get plenty of fluids when BG is high — our body will need them to help us not get dehydrated.

Bottom line: when you're sick, call your doctor to adjust your insulin doses just to be safe!

Reflection:
What we celebrate grows.

The things we fist pump and applaud are the things that flourish.
Who has been your biggest support this week?

_____

_____

_____

_____

_____

_____

_____

_____

_____

_____

_____

_____

_____

_____

_____

HOW DO WE TREAT HIGH BLOOD SUGAR?

If we have a stubborn high blood sugar level that we need to bring down, there are a few things that we can do to help. First — and the most obvious — is insulin! (Did you think I was gonna say Chuck Norris? Because I almost did.) Taking insulin and waiting about 30 minutes to an hour for it to kick in is the best and first thing to do. (Remember, it will take 3-4 hours for injectable rapid-acting insulin to fully correct a high blood sugar. Be patient. Don't "rage bolus" and take too much!)

While you're taking insulin and watching your levels, make sure to stay hydrated. Your body tries to get rid of any excess glucose in the bloodstream by peeing it out, and that's why frequent urination comes up a lot when talking about a high. The more water you drink, the more you can help flush out extra urine and rehydrate. You need to drink water — super important.

Checking for ketones is another vital response, and we'll talk about that in the next chapter.

Going for a light walk around the block is helpful if you're high because it increases how quickly your cells grab that glucose and get it into the cells that need it. In other words: exercise can help bring high blood sugar down faster. But if you have ketones, there's still too little insulin on board, and your BG is over 250 mg/dL, exercise can make things worse. Make sure you know what's going on before using exercise to help lower high BGs.

Reflection:
The highs and lows will happen, but it's what we do with the in-between moments that count!

Away from the anxious moments, the math, the medicine...what did you learn that will benefit you next week and next month?

_____

_____

_____

_____

_____

_____

_____

_____

_____

_____

_____

_____

_____

_____

WHAT ARE THE COMPLICATIONS OF
HIGH BLOOD SUGAR?

If your blood sugar levels stay elevated over a long period of time, it can have a drastic effect on your body. Not to mention that people get crabby when their blood sugar is high! My wife can tell when my blood sugar is high because my attitude goes right down the drain. I'm normally a positive person, but if my blood sugar is too high, all bets are off. (Sorry, Gina!)

Hyperglycemia can lead to many long-term complications:
- Kidney disease
- Heart disease
- Stroke
- Nerve damage
- Retinopathy

All diabetes complications start with damage to the blood vessels and nerve endings throughout every organ. Then, those organs fail to function properly. The best remedy for any of these is doing your best to keep your blood sugar levels in your target range — which is an endless, daily job.

Reflection:
Good habits must be established before they can be improved.

You're out there doing the hard work of balancing T1D and life! What is one thing that's working well for you?

_____

_____

_____

_____

_____

_____

_____

_____

_____

_____

_____

_____

_____

_____

WHAT IS INSULIN SENSITIVITY?

Everyone has different levels of "insulin sensitivity." Yours is different from mine and can/will change throughout your life. It can change quickly and slowly.

Insulin sensitivity determines how much insulin our body needs. Some things can make you more sensitive to insulin, meaning you'd need less insulin to keep your blood sugars in your target range. Other things can make you more resistant — which means you'd need more insulin to keep your blood sugars in your target range.

There are a bunch of things outside our control that lower our insulin sensitivity.
- Diet (eating less/more, improving choices, etc.)
- Physical activity (exercising more/less)
- Weight gain vs. weight loss (even just 5 pounds!)
- Hormones (growth, menstruation, menopause)
- Stress (short and long-term changes in stress)

One of the best things you can do to improve how sensitive you are to insulin (which is a good thing) is exercise. Something simple, like going for a walk every day, helps your body respond better to insulin overall.

Reflection:
The old you isn't the new you.

Today is brand new, and so are you! You're wiser for having gone through yesterday and learned something. Name one area that you've grown the most.

_____

_____

_____

_____

_____

_____

_____

_____

_____

_____

_____

_____

_____

_____

_____

CHAPTER 7

What is DKA?

Scan this before you start reading Chapter 7.

A lot of people, when they're first diagnosed with T1D, go into DKA. DKA means diabetic ketoacidosis. It's the big bad wolf.

MY HISTORY WITH DKA

When you develop moderate-to-large amounts of ketones in your blood, it shocks your body — basically, system failure.

A few things that combine to cause DKA are:
- Lack of insulin
- Continued high blood sugars — if you're over 300 mg/dL for a long time
- Severe dehydration — sometimes caused by vomiting
- Everyday illness, like the flu

I have gone into DKA three times in my life.
1. When I was first diagnosed in the Air Force. I was sick for about three months and didn't know the warning signs. When I finally went to the emergency room, my blood sugar was 1800 mg/dL. (This isn't a competition.)
2. When I had the flu, I couldn't keep food down, wasn't getting enough water, and my body shut down. The stress of the virus led to the development of ketones. (I didn't know back then that calling my doctor and adjusting my basal insulin could've probably prevented those ketones!)
3. Just a dumb error on my part; my blood was too high for too long, and I wasn't getting enough insulin.

Reflection:
Be honest with yourself about how you're feeling today.

Take a minute and breathe in how you feel, without judgment. What can you be honest about that maybe you've been tiptoeing around before?

_____

_____

_____

_____

_____

_____

_____

_____

_____

_____

_____

_____

_____

_____

WHAT ARE THE WARNING SIGNS OF DKA?

Insulin is a hormone that transforms glucose from the food we eat into energy for the body. When the body doesn't have enough insulin, it can lead to T1D symptoms. DKA is often misidentified as other conditions but can be extremely dangerous.

Symptoms like these are sometimes misinterpreted as a urinary tract infection, growth spurts in children and teenagers, type 2 diabetes, an eating disorder or other medical conditions. DKA can be confused for the flu, COVID-19, or a stomach virus.

Remember, the immediate symptoms of high blood sugar include:
- Sudden irritability
- Cravings (even if you just ate)
- Sudden drowsiness
- Headache
- Thirst
- Difficulty concentrating

And it can look like mood swings or irritability, waking up at night to get water or frequent trips to the bathroom.

Reflection:
Nobody remembers "easy".

What you're doing in managing T1D is memorable and noteworthy!
It takes a lot of hard work. What is one thing that you can learn
from today?

_____

_____

_____

_____

_____

_____

_____

_____

_____

_____

_____

_____

_____

_____

CAUSES OF DKA

Diabetic ketoacidosis (DKA) is a severe condition that can potentially lead to diabetic coma or even death. It occurs when excessive amounts of ketones are present in the blood.

DKA occurs when there is too little insulin available in your bloodstream. It can develop:
- In the weeks and months before your diagnosis
- If you forget to take your insulin
- If your insulin pump malfunctions and doesn't deliver insulin properly
- If your insulin is damaged (like, by extreme temperatures) and thus no potent
- If you come down with "regular people sickness" like the flu
- If you vomit excessively due to a stomach virus (severe dehydration)
- and more!

DKA gets treated in the hospital, but we can help prevent it by testing for ketones and checking our blood sugar on a regular basis! Don't try to manage DKA at home — your body needs more fluids to rebalance than you could possibly drink! (And you can't get everything you need from water!)

Reflection:
Every day is day one.

The door is shut on yesterday, and you've got a brand new day ahead of you! What is one area that you've grown most in?

_____

_____

_____

_____

_____

_____

_____

_____

_____

_____

_____

_____

_____

_____

HOW DO WE CHECK FOR KETONES?

DKA can happen when we're first diagnosed OR in the day-to-day management of T1D. So, what are the ways we can do our best to make sure we don't go there? (I kinda treat DKA like "he who shall not be named")

If you think you're in danger of DKA — check your ketones.
You can buy ketone strips at any drug store, online or anywhere for about $12. You pee on it, wait about 15 seconds, and it'll tell you if you've got ketones in your system based on the color results.

The other way is to get a blood ketone test kit from Amazon for about $50. These look almost exactly like a regular glucometer, but these test for ketones. You prick your finger, put it in the meter, and it'll give you a number.

Under 0.6	You're fine
0.6 to 1.5	Slight risk, maybe check again in a couple of hours
1.6 to 2.9	You're not in the danger zone, but you're on the highway to it
3 or higher	Go to the hospital or doctor right away

Reflection:

You're not doing a bad job; you're doing a difficult job.

Numbers are just numbers — not "good or bad." What is something you can celebrate that you did well today?

_____

_____

_____

_____

_____

_____

_____

_____

_____

_____

_____

_____

_____

_____

IS THERE TREATMENT FOR DKA?

When you go into DKA, your body gets all out of whack because you depleted your supply of minerals and chemicals as you fight to lower your blood sugar. This means your levels are dangerously low, and it's called an Anion Gap.

A normal anion gap is the difference between our proteins, organic acids, phosphates, and the potassium, calcium and magnesium levels. That may sound weird, but if we go into the hospital, the doctors aren't simply trying to lower our blood sugars.

If you go into DKA and go to the hospital's emergency department, here's what you can expect:

- You'll need intravenous fluids (which means setting up an IV in a vein in your arm). The fluids contain saline, potassium, and chloride. These fluids help flush out the ketones while rebalancing your bloodstream.
- Intravenous insulin is next. This isn't always included — it depends on the cause of your DKA and the severity.
- How long will you be there? It depends on what got you there. A little bit of vomiting and a 24-hour stomach bug means you might leave after one day. Severe DKA can require a longer stay.
- Depending on the severity and cause of your DKA, you might get some other tests done to check on the health and safety of other organs, including your kidneys and brain.

While going to the hospital is never fun, getting to the ER is imperative if you suspect you're in DKA or approaching DKA. If you're vomiting and can't keep fluids down, going to the ER is a must!

Reflection:

We are building resilience in us! We're stronger for it and more capable than we ever knew!

Resilience is our superpower, living with T1D. It's building muscles in us that we would never think to work out! What is one thing you can do for yourself today?

_____

_____

_____

_____

_____

_____

_____

_____

_____

_____

_____

_____

_____

_____

SICK DAYS AND DKA

One of the ways we can get blindsided by DKA is a common cold or flu. When we fight a viral infection, our blood sugar levels can get dangerously high, and keeping fluids or food down can be challenging. That can lead to dehydration, and before you know it, you've got a recipe for disaster! Here are a few things that most doctors agree on when it comes to developing a "sick day plan" and being on the lookout for DKA symptoms.

- Stay hydrated with clear broths or clear drinks without caffeine
- Drink plenty of electrolytes from zero-sugar sports drinks like Gatorade Zero
- Stock up on ketone strips to test regularly
- Call your doctor if your BG is over 240 mg/dL

Keep in mind that taking some cold and flu medications can elevate our blood sugars, so you may need to take more insulin than usual. If your doctor prescribes a steroid shot, it will most likely raise your BG for the day or even longer.

The rule of thumb on hydration is to drink 8 oz of water, zero-sugar sports drinks or clear broth every hour. That may sound like a lot, but the alternative is getting dehydrated, and that's bad news, kid! (read this last sentence in Chris Pratt's voice from Guardians of the Galaxy)

Reflection:
What we celebrate grows.

The things we fist pump and applaud are the things that flourish. Who has been your biggest support this week?

_____

_____

_____

_____

_____

_____

_____

_____

_____

_____

_____

_____

_____

COMMON MISCONCEPTIONS ABOUT DKA

You may be thinking, "Did we really need to spend an entire chapter on DKA, Neil?" The answer is a resounding heck yes, we did! This is so deadly, and there is a reason so many T1D organizations spend most of their time educating and advocating for the early warning signs of DKA. Here are a few facts that may shock you!

- You can have DKA even if your BG is only around 250 mg/dL. So many times, we think that it only happens when we have crazy high levels in the 800s, but that's not true.
- Ketones aren't the only symptom of DKA. The combination of a lot of different symptoms can throw you off, so be on the lookout for nausea, fevers or abdominal pain.
- Just because someone is in DKA doesn't mean their BG is out of control. It can happen due to an infection or flu that's out of our control.
- Insulin is only part of the remedy to DKA! It takes a lot of fluids, potassium and electrolytes to bring our levels back to normal.

Please remember the signs of DKA and remember that it's a sneaky little bugger. Even if you slightly suspect that DKA may be happening, check for ketones right away!

Reflection:
The highs and lows will happen, but it's what we do with the in-between moments that count!

Away from the anxious moments, the math, the medicine...what did you learn that will benefit you next week and next month?

_____

_____

_____

_____

_____

_____

_____

_____

_____

_____

_____

_____

_____

CHAPTER 8

Things that affect our BG

Scan this before you start reading Chapter 8.

Everybody tells us just to eat healthy foods and go for a walk, and we'll be right as rain! Turns out there's a whole lot more going on.

WHAT ARE THE 42 FACTORS THAT AFFECT BLOOD GLUCOSE?

You may be familiar with the organization "Diatribe" — a super helpful, knowledgeable, and solid nonprofit website and team over there.

Back in 2014, Adam Brown published a list called "22 factors that affect our blood glucose" for Diatribe. And you may be thinking, 22 doesn't sound like a lot. You're right — there are so many more than that. And in typical fashion, the diabetes community petitioned them with thousands of recommendations. And so, the list was updated to 42 factors that affect blood glucose.

You're counting in your head right now, aren't you?! I don't know about you, but juggling food, exercise, and medicine is hard enough! Everybody tells us just to eat healthy foods and go for a walk, and we'll be right as rain! Turns out there's a whole lot more going on.

Reflection:
Good habits must be established before they can be improved.

You're out there doing the hard work of balancing T1D and life! What is one thing that's working well for you?

_____

_____

_____

_____

_____

_____

_____

_____

_____

_____

_____

_____

_____

_____

WHAT RAISES BLOOD GLUCOSE?

We're going to throw things into two categories: "raises our BG" or "lowers our BG." Because, let's be honest, very few things out there have zero effect on your blood sugar.

Carbohydrates: The rule of thumb is "all carbohydrates count." It doesn't matter if you're eating low-carb, high-carb, keto, paleo, vegan, or you eat like a Hufflepuff at the Christmas Ball — carbs matter. Carbs get broken down into glucose in your digestive system and then into your bloodstream.

Protein: It should be mentioned that even though protein doesn't affect your BG as much as carbs, it can still require some careful insulin dosing. When you eat large amounts of protein (like a giant hamburger or a steak), your body only needs so many amino acids, so it converts the extra protein into glucose! It's still a slow impact on your blood sugar, but it's worth paying attention to.

Dietary fat: Just like protein, dietary fat matters, too. Fat doesn't raise BG, but it blunts your sensitivity to insulin and slows the digestion of the carbs in the meal. If you're eating a meal with a lot of fat (particularly saturated fat, like butter, bacon, cheese, etc.), you'll notice the impact of the meal on your blood sugar can take hours longer than lower fat meals. Pizza, for example, can take 6-8 hours to digest, which means you need to spread your insulin dose out more carefully.

Reflection:
The old you isn't the new you.

Today is brand new, and so are you! You're wiser for having gone through yesterday and learned something. Name one area that you've grown the most.

_____

_____

_____

_____

_____

_____

_____

_____

_____

_____

_____

_____

_____

WHAT ELSE RAISES BLOOD GLUCOSE?

Alcohol: Yes, alcohol can raise or lower your blood glucose. Here's why alcohol can be tricky for people with diabetes: it interferes with your liver's role in managing your blood sugar. When you drink alcohol, your liver focuses on processing and getting rid of the alcohol instead of releasing its usual drip, drip, drip of stored glucose. If you go to bed with a lot of alcohol in your system, you run the risk of running low in the later hours when you're not eating. You may have insulin on board, and your liver isn't releasing normal amounts of glucose.

Caffeine: It's proven science — caffeine triggers a hormonal response in your body that can raise blood sugar levels. First, it blocks adenosine receptors, which increases cell activity. Then, it increases the release of adrenaline, which signals the liver to release stored glucose into the bloodstream. Some people can have several cups of coffee before seeing a rise in BG; others may see an impact after only one cup. Everybody's sensitivity to caffeine is a little different. But if you're chugging coffee all day, don't be surprised if you're struggling with what seems like insulin resistance, too. Chances are, all the caffeine is telling your liver to release a lot of glucose all day. (A good reason to manage your caffeine consumption!)

Meal Timing: Skipping breakfast can actually cause your blood sugar to spike in the morning. This happens because your liver says, 'Well, you're not gonna feed your body fuel to get going, so I'm gonna release some stored glucose for fuel instead.' This isn't necessarily a bad thing, but it is something you'll have to anticipate if you skip breakfast or practice intermittent fasting.

Reflection:
Be honest with yourself about how you're feeling today.

Take a minute and breathe in how you feel, without judgment. What can you be honest about that maybe you've been tiptoeing around before?

THERE'S MORE THAT RAISES MY BLOOD GLUCOSE?

Steroids: Corticosteroids are medications used to treat asthma, rashes, arthritis, or sore joints. Topical creams or inhalable steroids don't seem to affect blood glucose, but the steroids that come in pills or injections raise your blood sugar and can last 3 to 10 days.

Niacin: Niacin is vitamin B3 and has been studied for its effects on managing lipids, and it's super helpful. However, a clinical trial of around 8300 people called the Coronary Drug Project showed that it significantly raised blood glucose levels.

Too little sleep: A study in the National Library of Medicine called Diabetes Care found that one night a week of only four hours of sleep can lower your insulin sensitivity by up to 21 percent! In other words, not enough sleep = insulin resistance. That means getting enough snooze time is extra important for people living with T1D.

Reflection:
Nobody remembers "easy".

What you're doing in managing T1D is memorable and noteworthy! It takes a lot of hard work. What is one thing that you can learn from today?

_____

_____

_____

_____

_____

_____

_____

_____

_____

_____

_____

_____

_____

_____

OH COME ON, THIS RAISES MY BLOOD GLUCOSE, TOO?

Dawn Phenomenon: This will raise our blood sugars, which happens in people with and without diabetes! This happens in your body anywhere between 2 AM and 8 AM. Your body releases hormones like cortisol, growth hormone, and adrenaline to "get us going in the morning," which tells the liver to release glucose throughout, effectively raising blood sugar levels.

Allergies: Dust, pollen, animals, and different foods all cause your body to react whether you want it to or not. One of the side effects of allergic reactions is your body gets dehydrated. The reason your blood sugar rises isn't directly connected to the allergy itself but some of the symptoms of allergies themselves.

Sunburn: A decent sunburn can raise blood sugar because it's essentially an injury to the body. Injury triggers inflammation, which leads to insulin resistance. Your body has to heal that burnt skin, kind of like the insulin resistance you experience when your body is fighting off a virus. It's a big stressor on the body. Sunburn also comes with a bit of dehydration, which increases the amount of sugar in your blood because you've decreased the water. Drink up and wear your sunscreen!

Reflection:
Every day is day one.

The door is shut on yesterday, and you've got a brand new day ahead of you! What is one area that you've grown most in?

_____

_____

_____

_____

_____

_____

_____

_____

_____

_____

_____

_____

_____

_____

WHAT LOWERS MY BLOOD GLUCOSE?

Light exercise: The American Diabetes Association tested the effects of light exercise on our blood sugars after a meal. This could be chores around the house, yard work or a walk that's not strenuous. They found that it cut the need for insulin almost in half for people with diabetes and those without it! Even a steady walk after eating can lead to severe hypoglycemia if you don't reduce the insulin dose for your meal. Light exercise can lower our BG! This can take a lot of trial and error. (Be sure to always keep fast-acting carbs, like juice or gummies, in your pocket when exercising!)

Intense exercise: Yeah, that CrossFit workout is intense, which is why it can actually spike your blood sugar. It's easy to assume that any heart-pounding workout will drop blood sugar, but anaerobic exercise (intense, short bursts of action) can trigger your body to create its own glucose! Learning the difference between aerobic and anaerobic exercise is a must!

Recent Hypoglycemia: When another low happens after you've recently had a low, it's harder to recognize symptoms, leading to an even more difficult time avoiding it. Dr. Philip Cryer studied 45 people living with T1D for 855 nights, and it's true. When you have a hypoglycemic event, you're more likely to have another one later because you can't feel or see it coming. Lows can deplete some of the stored glucose in your liver, which increases your risk for another low that same day because your liver glucose stores are low!

Reflection:
You're not doing a bad job; you're doing a difficult job.

Numbers are just numbers — not "good or bad." What is something you can celebrate that you did well today?

_____

_____

_____

_____

_____

_____

_____

_____

_____

_____

_____

_____

_____

_____

WHAT ELSE LOWERS MY BLOOD GLUCOSE?

Inaccurate BG reading: Getting an inaccurate blood glucose reading from a finger stick or our CGM can mess up everything. The National Library of Medicine says that when you check your blood, the test strip only needs 0.3 microliters of blood, and a speck of glucose on your finger the size of a dust particle can give a false reading by 300 mg/dl! It's pretty crucial that you don't inject insulin for a false reading!

Outside Temperature: The heat can make your blood sugar high or low. Heat can cause dehydration, and the glucose in your blood becomes more concentrated when there's less water. Heat also expands your blood vessels, which helps those cells pick up insulin and glucose. This increases your risk of hypoglycemia. The same effect happens in a hot tub, sauna or hot shower. While you're relaxing, keep an eye on your BG!

Celiac Disease: Anyone living with celiac disease will most likely be eating a gluten-free diet. If untreated, celiac disease can cause gastroparesis — a condition where the stomach empties too slowly. This delays how our food is digested & can lead to unpredictable levels.

Reflection:
We are building resilience in us! We're stronger for it and more capable than we ever knew!

Resilience is our superpower, living with T1D. It's building muscles in us that we would never think to work out! What is one thing you can do for yourself today?

_____

_____

_____

_____

_____

_____

_____

_____

_____

_____

_____

_____

_____

_____

CHAPTER 9

Food & Carbohydrates

Scan this before you start reading Chapter 9.

The moment you're diagnosed with any type of diabetes, your daily focus becomes food, food, food. And the 854 diets the internet is trying to sell you.

WHAT SHOULD WE OR SHOULDN'T WE EAT?

The moment you're diagnosed with any type of diabetes, your daily focus becomes food, food, food. What you "should" eat. What you "shouldn't" eat. What you want to eat. And the 854 diets the internet is trying to sell you.

I feel like I've tried everything in the last 31 years of living with T1D. I've eaten low-carb and tried Paleo. I have danced around with the Mediterranean Diet. I have been on keto for a few years as well. There's even a carnivore diet — which demands that you eat pretty much only meat — and I tried that, too!

Not to mention, in the first seven years of having T1D, I ate ANYTHING I WANTED!

I'm going to boil down my overall experience with diet and T1D. All the carbs count. Just count them. If you want them to be vegan carbs, spicy carbs, or only chili cheese coneys with crispy jalapeno carbs, count them. Because they count. None of us are getting away from that — so focus on what works for you and helps keep you healthy and your levels steady.

Reflection:
What we celebrate grows.

The things we fist pump and applaud are the things that flourish.
Who has been your biggest support this week?

_____

_____

_____

_____

_____

_____

_____

_____

_____

_____

_____

_____

_____

_____

WHAT HAPPENS TO OUR RELATIONSHIP WITH FOOD?

T1D can have a considerable impact on your relationship with food. How could it not? You have to think about every crumb you eat. You're under constant pressure to make perfect choices. It's a magical recipe for disordered eating.

Did you know that eating disorders are the second deadliest mental health condition in the US? It's alarming how chronic dieting and disordered eating have become everyday occurrences.

However, when we search for "relationship with food & T1D", most resources will only discuss standard ADA diets, low carb, paleo, or counting carbs—very few touch on how we can address the mental aspect of this issue.

To set the record straight — disordered eating isn't the same thing as an eating disorder. And it's more common than we may think. It could be cutting out entire food groups, labeling foods as good or bad, feeling guilty after eating certain foods, skipping meals on purpose, or constantly thinking about foods "we can't have."

If you've done this or thought this way — you're in good company. I have, too.

Reflection:

The highs and lows will happen, but it's what we do with the in-between moments that count!

Away from the anxious moments, the math, the medicine...what did you learn that will benefit you next week and next month?

_____

_____

_____

_____

_____

_____

_____

_____

_____

_____

_____

_____

_____

_____

BUILD A HEALTHY RELATIONSHIP WITH FOOD & DIABETES

Okay, I have a friend who is very passionate about this topic. Her name is Ginger Vieira and here she is: "Don't let diabetes turn you into a crazy diet monster. There's a lot of pressure to eat some insanely perfect diet when you're diagnosed with T1D. And most of us can't live with that pressure. Instead, we end up on this wild dieting yo-yo disaster where we try to be perfect for three weeks, then eat all the chocolate cake for a week, then rinse and repeat.

Yuck. It's exhausting. And unnecessary. Skip that drama and try this instead: don't try to be perfect. Instead, strive for an 80/20 approach to nutrition. For 80 percent of the day, you're trying to choose real food. That means fruit, nuts, animal protein (that hasn't been stuffed with cheesy sauce and wrapped in fried bread), grains, and veggies, veggies, veggies. If you need salad dressing on your salad, okay! No big deal! At least it helps get the salad down. The point is to choose mostly real food.

Then that leaves the 20 percent. It might be fries or pizza or chocolate. It's whatever helps you prevent feeling deprived. It's what helps you keep choosing those real foods the other 80 percent of the time. For example: You might find that eating lower carb during the day is helpful, but getting some yummy carbs at night keeps feelings of deprivation in check so you don't end up eating all the cookies and a whole box of cereal on Friday night.

Other helpful goals: ditch the diet soda and the diet products. (Water! Seltzer!) Take a closer look at how much alcohol you're drinking. And juice or soda? Juice and soda are all sugar, baby. Save your sugar for your 20 percent in something more worthwhile. How much coffee or Redbulls are you chugging?

Reflection:
Good habits must be established before they can be improved.

You're out there doing the hard work of balancing T1D and life! What is one thing that's working well for you?

_____

_____

_____

_____

_____

_____

_____

_____

_____

_____

_____

_____

_____

_____

WHAT ARE NET CARBS?

Today, we're talking about the ratio of fiber to total carbs and the form that the carb comes in.

First, fiber — and insert the Turd Furgeson jokes here. Fiber is our friend! Fiber is a carbohydrate that isn't digested. It slows digestion so our insulin can catch up. Foods with a high fiber have a lower impact on blood glucose than foods with the same amount of total carbs and no fiber.

So, load up on green veggies, nuts, or a low-carb/high-fiber tortilla, etc. The more whole foods you're eating, the more fiber you're getting. Eat more whole, real foods!

There's also something called net carbs. These are the amount of "impact carbs" in a food. But here's a funny thing to remember: a lot of this is about marketing. Some of the fiber can be broken down into glucose and can affect your blood sugar. The more a food product (versus a natural whole food) claims to contain a lot of fiber, the more likely it is a heavily processed manufactured fiber that will definitely affect your blood sugar.

Don't fall for the marketing. Don't eat a diet full of lousy diet products. Eat more real food. An apple with peanut butter is gonna offer you far more nutrition than some "keto peanut butter bar." Choose more real food.

Reflection:
The old you isn't the new you.

Today is brand new, and so are you! You're wiser for having gone through yesterday and learned something. Name one area that you've grown the most.

_____

_____

_____

_____

_____

_____

_____

_____

_____

_____

_____

_____

_____

_____

_____

WHAT ABOUT KETO, PALEO AND LOW CARB DIETS?

Many people living with T1D try eating a low-carb diet, a Paleo or a Keto diet at some point. Cutting carbs can be helpful, but that doesn't necessarily mean it's sustainable. If you can only follow a Keto diet for three weeks before eating all the carbs, then it's not actually a great fit for you.

Make sure you choose an approach to nutrition that you can stick to for the long haul. Sustainability is critical because if you can't stick with it, fall off the wagon, and binge eat, is the diet really helping you?

There's so much pressure to cut all the carbs. Part of thriving with T1D is learning how to dose insulin for carbs. You're not gonna do it perfectly all the time. It's okay.

There are some people who follow strict low-carb diets and thrive. It's really about a personality type, not a "this person is hardcore, and this person isn't." For most people, the degree of restriction isn't a great fit — and that's okay.

Reflection:

Be honest with yourself about how you're feeling today.

Take a minute and breathe in how you feel, without judgment. What can you be honest about that maybe you've been tiptoeing around before?

_____

_____

_____

_____

_____

_____

_____

_____

_____

_____

_____

_____

_____

_____

ARE SUGAR ALCOHOLS REALLY "FREE"?

The benefit of sugar alcohols is that for people living with T1D, they aren't fully absorbed or digested by your body. Good right? Not so fast!

Sugar alcohols are usually derived from fruit, and they don't break down into glucose like other carbohydrates do, which means they aren't supposed to impact your blood sugar as much. But it isn't quite this simple.

To spot sugar alcohols in your food, look at the nutrition label on the side, look under "total carbohydrates," and then under the category labeled "sugar alcohols." If you want to get specific, read the ingredients list to see exactly which kind of sugar alcohol is hiding in the food.

Sugar alcohols can lead to "explosive diarrhea" really fast! More politely, sugar alcohols can wreak havoc on your digestive system. Go read Amazon reviews of sugar-free gummy bears for the most descriptive and fascinatingly offensive play-by-play of the aftermath these things can have.

Most "sugar-free" gums, candies, and mints have around two calories per gram; according to the FDA, that's still under the 3 calories/gram limit. So it says "sugar-free," but if we eat a bunch of them, we'll still see an impact on our blood sugar.

Beware of the processed, low-carb diet products!

Reflection:
Nobody remembers "easy".

What you're doing in managing T1D is memorable and noteworthy! It takes a lot of hard work. What is one thing that you can learn from today?

_____

_____

_____

_____

_____

_____

_____

_____

_____

_____

_____

_____

_____

WHAT IS A "PRE-BOLUS" BEFORE A MEAL?

Are you tired of seeing your blood sugar spike after you eat? Yeah — me, too! Meeeeeee, too! Pre-bolus is simply taking insulin before eating to help your insulin get the jump on the food. Pre-bolusing gives insulin a head start before your food is digested. Here are a few things to keep in mind:

- Never pre-bolus for a meal if your blood sugar is low when you start eating.
- Never pre-bolus for a meal at a restaurant when you're not sure just how long it'll take for that food to show up.
- Never pre-bolus for a meal if you're hustling as a parent with little kids, and you might forget to eat your meal or get distracted because Little Jimmy threw his mac n' cheese at Little Lucy, and you won't be eating dinner until they finally go to bed.
- Never pre-bolus for a meal if you're taking inhaled insulin and are unfamiliar with how fast that meal hits your blood sugar.

How far ahead of your meal you want to pre-bolus depends on what you're eating, how much activity you've had before the meal and what kind of insulin you use. Most rapid-acting insulins take about 15 to 30 minutes to start working and peak at 1 hour. If you're taking rapid-acting inhaled insulin, that kicks in under 5 minutes and peaks at 30 minutes. For example, a regular ol' apple will digest pretty quickly. Your healthcare team would probably suggest a 15-minute pre-bolus, which means taking your insulin dose for the apple about 15 minutes before eating so it's already rolling in your bloodstream by the time the apple hits your bloodstream. Pre-bolusing is tedious. Lots of people don't bother. Lots of people try their best. Some people do it perfectly. This will probably take a little bit of time and experimentation to get it right, but it's a huge win when it works! Do your best. It's not easy.

Reflection:
Every day is day one.

The door is shut on yesterday, and you've got a brand new day ahead of you! What is one area that you've grown most in?

_____

_____

_____

_____

_____

_____

_____

_____

_____

_____

_____

_____

_____

_____

_____

CHAPTER 10

Exercise & Activity

Scan this before you start reading Chapter 10.

Fasted exercise is a straightforward way to encourage your body to burn fat for fuel instead of sugar from your bloodstream.

WHAT TYPES OF EXERCISE AFFECT BLOOD SUGAR?

Managing exercise with T1D can be challenging due to several factors, such as the type, duration, timing of the workout, the type of insulin used, and mode of delivery (pump or injections). Other variables, including the last time you ate, can also impact our blood sugar levels. There are two types of exercise, and you should know which you're doing when you head out for your next workout because they can impact your blood sugar very differently.

- Aerobic exercise like walking, running, hiking or even doing yard work can bring your blood sugar down quickly if you have "insulin on board" from a meal, a correction bolus, or simply too much basal/background insulin.
- Anaerobic exercise like weight lifting, CrossFit or any other high-intensity interval training can raise your blood sugar for several reasons. Mostly, it's due to your body converting lactic acid into glucose and releasing stored glucose from your liver to give you energy. In competitive sports, adrenaline can tell your liver to dump glucose, too. Even with too much insulin on board, though, anaerobic exercise can also cause your blood sugar to drop.

Many people find "fasted" exercise to be the simplest. This means you're exercising before you eat — when it's been at least 3 or 4 hours since your last meal — because that reduces how much insulin you'll have in your bloodstream during exercise. You may have to adjust your pump's basal rate, too.

Fasted exercise is a straightforward way to encourage your body to burn fat for fuel instead of sugar from your bloodstream. It'll take some trial and error, but once you get the hang of it, it can really help simplify exercising with T1D.

Reflection:
What we celebrate grows.

The things we fist pump and applaud are the things that flourish.
Who has been your biggest support this week?

_____

_____

_____

_____

_____

_____

_____

_____

_____

_____

_____

_____

_____

WHAT IF MY BLOOD SUGAR IS HIGH BEFORE I EXERCISE?

It's super important to bring down high blood sugars, especially when planning to exercise. However, you need to approach this with caution. To avoid a sudden drop in blood sugar levels, you can administer a lower insulin dose to bring your level within the desired range.

This way, we can still benefit from exercising on an empty stomach.

For example: to keep my blood sugar from rising during anaerobic workouts, I take ¼ units of Novolog if my blood sugar is 200 mg/dL. This is a 75% reduction from my usual 1-unit correction dose.

In other words: be very cautious when correcting high blood sugars before exercise because the exercise will increase how much glucose your cells pick up. This means you need far less insulin to correct that high than usual.

If your blood sugar level is above 250 mg/dL, there is a chance that exercise can lead to ketones and cause your blood sugar to rise further. It's important to be cautious when exercising with high blood sugar levels and ketones, as it can be dangerous. Best to wait until our ketones get to normal and our BG is closer to our target before doing a workout.

Reflection:
The highs and lows will happen, but it's what we do with the in-between moments that count!

Away from the anxious moments, the math, the medicine...what did you learn that will benefit you next week and next month?

_____

_____

_____

_____

_____

_____

_____

_____

_____

_____

_____

_____

_____

_____

_____

WHAT IF MY BLOOD SUGAR IS LOW
BEFORE I EXERCISE?

If your blood sugar is low because you have too much insulin on board, it's best to treat the low and wait for the insulin to leave your system before hitting the treadmill or weight bench.

If you're a little low or wake up feeling slightly low but still want to do fasted exercise, try treating the low with as few carbs as possible.

This isn't true "fasted" exercise because of the food intake; it can still be done with minimal risk of experiencing low blood sugar if you keep your carb consumption small enough to avoid a bolus.

If my blood sugar is around 70 mg/dLs before exercising, I'll eat a few Sunkist fruit gels that have 8 carbs each, and it'll bring me up close to the 100 mg/dL range so I can go workout and get ripped, shredded, and jaaaaaacked!

Treating a low with minimal carbs means you know there isn't much insulin on board that could continue to drive your blood sugar down further.

Reflection:

Good habits must be established before they can be improved.

You're out there doing the hard work of balancing T1D and life! What is one thing that's working well for you?

_____

_____

_____

_____

_____

_____

_____

_____

_____

_____

_____

_____

_____

_____

WHAT EXERCISES RAISE MY BLOOD GLUCOSE?

Typically, anaerobic exercises such as weightlifting, spinning, sprinting, or CrossFit can increase our blood sugar levels. This is relatively common, and we shouldn't think something is wrong. It can even happen if we haven't had anything to eat yet!

During these kinds of exercises, our body transforms lactic acid into glucose, a fancy term called gluconeogenesis. This gives us enough fuel to do the workout, but it also raises our blood sugars. Adrenaline tells our liver to release stored glucose, and that "fight or flight" mentality kicks in. All this extra glucose needs insulin, so be careful of those spikes.

Even if we skip breakfast to make sure we don't have a high blood sugar during exercise, our liver can release stored glucose — which causes a spike. We may need some insulin halfway through the workout! (Yup, this means fasted exercise can lead to high blood sugars. Take good notes! You might find you need a tiny bolus of insulin during your fasted window to manage that extra liver glucose.)

Reflection:

The old you isn't the new you.

Today is brand new, and so are you! You're wiser for having gone through yesterday and learned something. Name one area that you've grown the most.

_____

_____

_____

_____

_____

_____

_____

_____

_____

_____

_____

_____

_____

_____

WHAT SHOULD I DO BEFORE I EXERCISE?

Hardly anything about exercising or activity when we live with T1D can be left up to chance. Very rarely will I just "go for a run" without spending a few hours thinking about it or prepping for it.

Always take something with you to the gym or outside if you're going for a run / hike / walk. Honey Stingers, Cliff Shots, Glucose tabs, gels — all of it works! Something that's pure glucose and doesn't have a lot of extra fiber or ingredients that will slow down our body's ability to absorb the glucose.

Almost every insulin pump on the market now is equipped with an activity mode specifically for this reason! If we take the time to set this temporary activity mode, the insulin pump will raise our overall target range to be a little higher than usual.

Many people find they need a dramatic reduction in basal insulin starting at least an hour before the exercise. (That could be programming as much as a 75% reduction!) Remember, the insulin you get from 3 to 4 p.m. is what affects your blood sugar between 4 to 6 p.m. You cannot simply set a temp basal when you start exercising. You need to plan ahead.

This bump from 110-120 mg/dL to 140-160 mg/dL will help the insulin pump keep our BGs a little higher so we don't have those low moments. It's best to set this activity mode about an hour before the actual activity so it can begin to curb off that insulin so we don't have too much in our system when exercising.

Reflection:
Be honest with yourself about how you're feeling today.

Take a minute and breathe in how you feel, without judgment. What can you be honest about that maybe you've been tiptoeing around before?

_____

_____

_____

_____

_____

_____

_____

_____

_____

_____

_____

_____

_____

_____

WHAT ARE INTRAMUSCULAR INJECTIONS?

There's one thing that can almost guarantee a double arrow down, if you know what I mean — intramuscular insulin injections. This is when you inject insulin directly into muscle instead of body fat, which causes it to be absorbed into your bloodstream much more quickly. Right now, the FDA doesn't approve any intramuscular injections, but many people use this for a few different reasons.

If you inject insulin directly into muscle or even a part of your body that doesn't have a lot of fat — you're at risk of hypoglycemia. And it will most likely sting a little when it hits your muscle.

If you don't want to risk this, try rubbing the area where you just gave an injection, take a hot shower or bath. I'm not rich — I don't have a hot tub or sauna, but that'll work too. The heat gets our blood flowing and moves the insulin around faster. Even exercise right after an injection in the legs will most likely give us a much faster response from the insulin.

Reflection:
Every day is day one.

The door is shut on yesterday, and you've got a brand new day ahead of you! What is one area that you've grown most in?

_____

_____

_____

_____

_____

_____

_____

_____

_____

_____

_____

_____

_____

_____

_____

_____

CHAPTER 11

Technology, Pumps & CGMs

Scan this before you start reading Chapter 11.

Only about 20 years ago, we dreamed of having an insulin pump that wasn't as big as carry-on luggage!

ARE WE LIVING IN THE GOLDEN AGE OF T1D TECH?

Right now, we have more diabetes tech, gadgets, connectivity and help than we've ever had in the past! Only about 20 years ago, we dreamed of having an insulin pump that wasn't as big as carry-on luggage!

With the advancements in islet cell research, reversing the damage to our pancreas, and early detection of T1D in family members, we're so much better off. (By the way, islet cells are the cells that contain beta cells, which are the cells produced by your pancreas that produce insulin!)

Most of the world doesn't have access to continuous glucose monitors (CGM) or insulin pumps, so if you have one, consider yourself blessed! This technology has allowed us to spend more time in range, which cuts down on your risk of T1D complications.

That's what we're all after, right? We don't want the effects of this disease to slow us down, delay our plans, or deviate our dreams, and that's why we're going to spend a chapter talking about some of the best new diabetes tech out there.

Time to nerd out!

Reflection:
You're not doing a bad job; you're doing a difficult job.

Numbers are just numbers — not "good or bad." What is something you can celebrate that you did well today?

_____
_____
_____
_____
_____
_____
_____
_____
_____
_____
_____
_____
_____
_____

WHAT ARE OUR OPTIONS WITH CGMS?

Continuous Glucose Monitors (CGM) are a pretty fantastic tool for managing diabetes. CGMs may look slightly different on the outside, but their basic function is pretty much the same. Here are some of the main CGMs on the market:

- Dexcom G6 or G7
- Abbott Freestyle Libre
- Medtronic Guardian 3
- Senseonics Eversence

In 1999, Minimed introduced the first CGM system, but it required SO MANY calibrations and you couldn't see the data in real-time. The next major improvement was in 2004 when Medtronic Guardian brought in wireless transmission and programmable glucose alerts. Medtronic Guardian RT and Dexcom STS were launched in 2005 and 2006, allowing patients to view their glucose levels in real-time for up to three days.

Most CGMs today give updated readings every 5 minutes, are wirelessly connected to a phone or device through Bluetooth connectivity, and we can see Time in Range and Standard Deviation on the fly. This gives us a chance to see what our estimated A1C is, and we don't have to wait to see the doctor. The peace of mind that a CGM brings is an absolute game-changer!

Reflection:

We are building resilience in us! We're stronger for it and more capable than we ever knew!

Resilience is our superpower, living with T1D. It's building muscles in us that we would never think to work out! What is one thing you can do for yourself today?

_____

_____

_____

_____

_____

_____

_____

_____

_____

_____

_____

_____

_____

_____

ARE CGMS ACCURATE?

In short, yes — but don't get all frazzled when the number on your CGM doesn't match your blood glucose monitor. They're not supposed to match.

CGMs actually measure the glucose in your interstitial fluid (ISF), which is the fluid in your fatty tissue. This is very different than measuring a blood glucose level because the glucose hits your bloodstream before it arrives in your ISF. So there's about a 15-minute delay between the two if your glucose level is actively fluctuating at that moment you're comparing.

Here's how it works: think of your blood as the highway of your body. It transfers glucose to your whole body while the fluid under your skin transfers it to the cells in your tissue. This is the rest stop on the highway in your body.

Doctors and scientists learned how to calculate what we call "the lag." This is the time between when your blood glucose reading is higher or lower than what the interstitial fluid showed. And don't get me wrong, the interstitial fluid eventually got to the same reading the blood showed; it was just slower. This lag or delay is vital to remember when we're doing an activity or exercising!

Reflection:
What we celebrate grows.

The things we fist pump and applaud are the things that flourish.
Who has been your biggest support this week?

_____

_____

_____

_____

_____

_____

_____

_____

_____

_____

_____

_____

_____

WHAT IS THE HISTORY OF INSULIN PUMPS?

The first insulin pump was invented in 1963. This thing was as big as a microwave and extremely expensive. In 1979, the first commercial insulin pump was made. Still stupidly expensive. And finally, in 1985, the first insulin pen, called the Novopen, was invented.

The insulin pump market is valued today at just under five billion dollars in the US alone and is projected to grow by almost 9% every year for the next 10 years! The whole market is divided into two categories: tubeless pumps and tethered insulin pumps. What blew my mind is which companies are larger and which pumps are the most widely used.

Today's newest options include:
- Omnipod's 5
- Medtronic's 780G
- Tandem's tSlim
- Beta Bionic's iLet
- AccuCheck's Solo

There are so many quality insulin pumps to choose from, and I highly recommend finding the one that works best for you. The pump you will use, learn about, understand and feel connected to is such a personal choice!

Reflection:
Good habits must be established before they can be improved.

You're out there doing the hard work of balancing T1D and life! What is one thing that's working well for you?

_____

_____

_____

_____

_____

_____

_____

_____

_____

_____

_____

_____

_____

_____

WHAT IS A HYBRID CLOSE-LOOP PUMP?

If you had an insulin pump before 2020, you'd remember that they simply delivered insulin based on a lot of manual programming, manual dosing for meals, and manual corrections for highs.

These pumps weren't connected to a CGM and were based more on convenience. You didn't need to take as many shots, which was a big plus. But it was kind of like getting strapped into a roller coaster — even if you didn't want the ride.

Because they operated off of pre-programmed basal rates, if your blood glucose dropped low at night, the pump would still give you insulin because it was programmed to do it. It wasn't able to make decisions based on blood glucose levels.

In these situations, their convenience wore off, and they weren't all that helpful, more harmful, actually. This is why the interconnectivity between a CGM and the pump became so important. These pumps are now called Automated Insulin Delivery systems (AID) — also known as "closed-loop pumps" because they do a lot of the thinking for you.

AID systems work with compatible pumps and CGMs that talk to each other. The pump is programmed with a highly complex algorithm that automatically adjusts your basal and bolus doses based on real-time data from your CGM. These AID systems can dramatically improve your time-in-range, decrease the hour-by-hour work of managing insulin, and ideally prevent severe lows and highs. They aren't perfect, but they can help a lot.

Currently, four major insulin pump manufacturers are taking up most of the market: Tandem, Omnipod, Medtronic, and AccuCheck.

Reflection:

The old you isn't the new you.

Today is brand new, and so are you! You're wiser for having gone through yesterday and learned something. Name one area that you've grown the most.

_____

_____

_____

_____

_____

_____

_____

_____

_____

_____

_____

_____

_____

_____

ARE THERE DUAL HORMONE PUMPS?

Beta Bionics is still working on the first "dual-hormone pump" approved to administer insulin and glucagon. This means the pump could treat lows in addition to highs and prevent impending lows. (Remember, glucagon is that hormone that tells your liver to release stored glucose!)

Imagine that most closed-loop pumps right now have a gas pedal. If you want to lower your blood glucose when it's high, you can slowly push the insulin in like you'd press a gas pedal. But if you start to drop too fast, the pump doesn't really have a brake pedal to stop your blood sugar from dropping. It can only "coast" for a bit. But if your insulin pump also had glucagon and could stop you from going too low, that would be next-level stuff right there!

While Ed Damiano, CEO of Beta Bionics, set out to create this technology years ago, he had to wait for better glucagon options. Until recently, glucagon was only stable for 24 hours, then expired. Today's modern glucagon options (glucagon has a much better shelf-life) mean Damiano and his team can begin human trials with their dual-hormone pump.

Reflection:
Be honest with yourself about how you're feeling today.

Take a minute and breathe in how you feel, without judgment. What can you be honest about that maybe you've been tiptoeing around before?

_____

_____

_____

_____

_____

_____

_____

_____

_____

_____

_____

_____

_____

_____

HOW DO CLOSED-LOOP PUMPS WORK?

Closed-loop pumps (or AID) systems work based on highly complex algorithms designed carefully by very smart-pants engineers. Each pump comes with its own algorithm.

The algorithm is designed to predict where your blood glucose will be in relation to how many carbohydrates you've eaten and how much insulin is on board. While these systems receive data every five minutes from your CGM, some AID systems can make changes up to a limited number of times per hour, depending on the brand.

The ability to slowly dial the amount of insulin back or up is a game changer. Prior to AID systems, insulin pumps were very similar to a light switch. The insulin was "on or off." Sure, we could set the amount of insulin you were getting, but there was very little in-the-moment fine-tuning.

Now, insulin pumps are more like a dimmer switch where you can slowly dial back or dial up the amount of insulin for a much smoother curve. Having these hybrid closed loops in place gives us so much more control and less decision fatigue!

Reflection:
Nobody remembers "easy".

What you're doing in managing T1D is memorable and noteworthy!
It takes a lot of hard work. What is one thing that you can learn
from today?

_____

_____

_____

_____

_____

_____

_____

_____

_____

_____

_____

_____

_____

_____

CHAPTER 12

Common Quirks & Questions

Scan this before you start reading Chapter 12.

Second, only in frustration to someone telling me that their cat also has diabetes, eye complications are one of the first things people think of with diabetes.

ARE COMPRESSION LOWS A PROBLEM WITH A CGM?

Sometimes at night, if you or someone in your family wearing a CGM has a low alert — you may think, "Oh, sheesh, wake them up and get them glucose." But there could be something else going on.

A compression low is a false reading caused simply by your body weight putting pressure on the CGM, usually when you're sleeping. Your blood sugar might not actually be low — but that's how the CGM interprets it. Here is what's really going on.

The CGM has a tiny metal filament that's inserted under the skin in your interstitial fluid. It doesn't read your blood glucose — it reads the glucose level in the fluid under your skin. This fluid surrounds your cells; when we squeeze that fluid, the CGM gives us an alarm!

This isn't a device error — it's your body "not delivering" enough fluid to the CGM sensor to perform accurately. That tiny metal filament needs fluid, and when it doesn't get it, we get an alarm.

Reflection:
Every day is day one.

The door is shut on yesterday, and you've got a brand new day ahead of you! What is one area that you've grown most in?

_____

_____

_____

_____

_____

_____

_____

_____

_____

_____

_____

_____

_____

_____

_____

_____

HOW DO I KNOW IF I'M IN A HONEYMOON PHASE?

Nope, it's not a shiny, sun-soaked trip to the Bahamas with the love of your life. When first diagnosed with T1D, your pancreas may still have a few beta cells hanging around that can produce insulin. That attack on your pancreas takes time, so while you're not producing enough insulin to stay out of the hospital, you're still producing some. When you start daily insulin therapy, it can actually take some of the pressure off your pancreas, and you start producing more insulin. And that's when the honeymoon begins!

Your body needs less insulin than usual, and your blood sugar may be easier to manage. Sounds great, right? Smoke and mirrors, my friends!

The honeymoon phase is temporary and unpredictable. How much insulin you're still making and for how long is different for everyone. And not everyone with T1D has a honeymoon period. People diagnosed during adulthood tend to have much longer honeymoon periods than children.

Regardless, you'll still need to make constant adjustments in your insulin doses and be super careful to monitor blood sugar levels. And when the honeymoon is over, it can be a little startling because your blood sugar can fluctuate much more dramatically without the help of your pancreas. You're not failing. This is part of T1D. Work with your healthcare team to continuously fine-tune your doses!

So embrace the honeymoon phase for what it is — a relatively short part of the journey.

Reflection:

You're not doing a bad job; you're doing a difficult job.

Numbers are just numbers — not "good or bad." What is something you can celebrate that you did well today?

_____

_____

_____

_____

_____

_____

_____

_____

_____

_____

_____

_____

_____

_____

WHAT IS RETINOPATHY?

Second, only in frustration to someone telling me that their cat also has diabetes, eye complications are one of the first things people think of with diabetes.

Diabetic retinopathy is caused by chronic hyperglycemia — that's high blood sugar along with genetics. The blood vessels in the back of your eyes are tiny, and if your blood sugars are too high for too long, you will get these little swelling spots called microaneurysms. They look like little tiny bubbles along the blood vessel. These swelling spots in the back of your eyes stop the blood flow to your retina, and the retina starts to secrete other chemicals, trying to get the blood vessels to grow new routes.

This fluid in the back of your eye makes the blood vessels bleed, scar tissue forms, and the retina detaches from the tissue, like pulling a sticker off the page.

The Cincinnati Eye Institute said the significant risk factors for developing diabetic retinopathy are "how long we've had the disease, poor sugar control and high blood pressure."

But tight blood sugar levels don't mean you can avoid annual eye exams. You should get your eyes checked with a dilated eye exam every year because you can treat and prevent vision loss if you catch retinopathy early! Regardless of blood sugar levels, anyone can develop mild-to-moderate retinopathy after many years of T1D. Get your eyes checked, baby! Every year.

Reflection:

We are building resilience in us! We're stronger for it and more capable than we ever knew!

Resilience is our superpower, living with T1D. It's building muscles in us that we would never think to work out! What is one thing you can do for yourself today?

_____

_____

_____

_____

_____

_____

_____

_____

_____

_____

_____

_____

_____

_____

_____

AM I INSULIN RESISTANT?

Your body's sensitivity to insulin can change wildly over the course of weeks and months. The more sensitive you are to insulin, the less you need in order to stay in range. The more resistant you are to insulin, the more you need to stay in range. Ideally, we want to be insulin sensitive and combat insulin resistance as much as possible through lifestyle habits.

Losing weight plays a significant role in your insulin sensitivity. Body fat blunts your sensitivity to insulin. Even losing 5 pounds will help — and can mean you need to reduce your basal and/or bolus insulin doses.

Daily exercise, even gentle walking, plays a huge role in your body's sensitivity to insulin because it increases how much glucose your cells take up. Daily exercise can change your insulin sensitivity throughout the entire day. If you suddenly start exercising every day, you'll definitely need to reduce all of your insulin doses! This is a good thing. Consistency counts. Exercise daily.

Getting more sleep! If you stay up late playing CALL OF DUTY until 2 AM, I promise it will show up in your blood sugars. If we don't get enough sleep, cortisol levels rise, which blunts our sensitivity to insulin. Insulin resistance can last up to 24 hours after staying up. Aim for 8 hours of sleep.

Drinking alcohol is something our body internally sees as a threat. And our liver doesn't work as well, which leads to insulin resistance. Especially binge drinking — a major no-no. But even just drinking every night of the week can greatly impact your insulin sensitivity. Let the tasty liquids be a treat, not a daily habit.

Reflection:
What we celebrate grows.

The things we fist pump and applaud are the things that flourish. Who has been your biggest support this week?

_____

_____

_____

_____

_____

_____

_____

_____

_____

_____

_____

_____

_____

_____

WHAT'S THE DIFFERENCE BETWEEN INSULIN STACKING AND RAGE BOLUS?

There are stubborn high blood sugars that sometimes we just can't seem to get to come down! Inevitably, we give a little insulin and wait, maybe not as long as we should because we're obsessing over every minute that goes by, and we don't see our number decrease! And so what happens?

Cue the Rage Bolus. A rage bolus is when you take an extra large dose of insulin, hoping to bring the high blood sugar down faster. But taking more insulin doesn't change how quickly it works.

Stacking insulin is another tricky mess. This is when, for example, you take insulin at 4 p.m., then again at 3:30 p.m., and so on. Now you have insulin-on-board peaking at different times, and it can easily result in severe lows.

I've done this. So many of us have done this! Because it can be challenging to sit back and wait while you feel the pain and guilt of a high blood sugar level, and you want to "speed the process up" but only make it worse.

In this situation, the best thing to do is wait, set a timer for an hour, and remember that most insulins take about 30 minutes before they start to kick in and hit their peak after an hour.

.

Reflection:
The highs and lows will happen, but it's what we do with the in-between moments that count!

Away from the anxious moments, the math, the medicine...what did you learn that will benefit you next week and next month?

_____

_____

_____

_____

_____

_____

_____

_____

_____

_____

_____

_____

_____

_____

_____

WHAT DO C-PEPTIDE AND AUTOANTIBODY TESTS DETERMINE?

When a healthy pancreas produces insulin, it makes equal amounts of c-peptides. Insulin is the hormone that helps regulate your blood sugar, and c-peptide is like its plus one. If you're making insulin, you're also making c-peptide. This test tells doctors whether or not you're making any insulin or if you're not making enough insulin. Doctors can tell what type of diabetes you have based on these test results. If you're producing plenty of c-peptide, that might mean your body has become insulin resistant, which means type 2 diabetes, not type 1.

A normal result typically falls between 0.5 ng/mL to 2.0 ng/mL or 0.17 to 0.83 nmol/L. A lower number could mean we're not making enough insulin; a high number could mean insulin resistance. These tests can also be a way to screen for kidney failure, pancreatic tumors or Cushing syndrome.

Autoantibodies, on the other hand, are the result of your immune system attacking your own body. Research has identified T1D-specific autoantibodies, and you can test for them! Here's what we know about autoantibodies:
- Most people develop autoantibodies years before having high blood sugars or symptoms.
- Most people have autoantibodies present before they're five years old even if you don't develop T1D symptoms until your teens, 20s, or beyond!
- Your family members can (and should) get tested for T1D autoantibodies by visiting TrialNet.org.
- If you test positive, you can potentially delay the need for insulin with teplizumab — an FDA-approved therapy that slows down the attack on your pancreas.

Reflection:

The old you isn't the new you.

Today is brand new, and so are you! You're wiser for having gone through yesterday and learned something. Name one area that you've grown the most.

_____

_____

_____

_____

_____

_____

_____

_____

_____

_____

_____

_____

_____

_____

IS FROZEN SHOULDER COMMON WITH T1D?

There's a very real thing called frozen shoulder that people living with T1D can develop. I'm not making this up! Frozen shoulder is super painful, making it difficult for people to move their arms and shoulders around. It would definitely prevent us from doing the Carlton.

The reason people with diabetes are at risk for this is that extra glucose in your body attaches to the collagen in your joints. Collagen is the protein that makes your joints move easier and holds them together. Extra sugar makes it sticky — think of any time you get syrup or something sugary on your hands. Over time, that collagen gets tougher and starts to harden. This can take months to set in, but there are ways to get that range of motion back.

Physical therapy and working on stretches to slowly improve that range of motion can help — it's what doctors call the "Thawing Stage." Massage can help, too, or you can get a steroid shot in the joint. That one can be super painful, and the steroids mess with your blood sugars for a bit. (Steroids can cause some mega insulin resistance!)

Reflection:
Be honest with yourself about how you're feeling today.

Take a minute and breathe in how you feel, without judgment.
What can you be honest about that maybe you've been tiptoeing
around before?

_____

_____

_____

_____

_____

_____

_____

_____

_____

_____

_____

_____

_____

_____

CHAPTER 13

Diabetes Burnout

Scan this before you start reading Chapter 13.

Like, be honest with yourself for a minute. T1D is a lot! It's okay to get rattled by this thing because you're carrying a lot. That's just the truth.

WHY DO I FEEL OVERWHELMED?

Every day you deal with T1D is a constant juggling of stuff you do to survive. And to be honest, I struggle with it all sometimes. You may struggle, too. And please hear me when I say this: it is okay to deal with this stuff. You're not doing anything wrong. You're not weak because of it. You're not alone in it.

Like, be honest with yourself for a minute. T1D is a lot! It's okay to get rattled by this thing because you're carrying a lot. That's just the truth. You carry so many daily decisions that can hit us emotionally and physically.

Dr. Mark said something in his book, "Diabetes Sucks and You Can Handle It" that really stuck with me.

"Diabetes isn't always going to make sense. That's just how it is, which is a big part of what makes diabetes so stressful."

He's right! Most days, it doesn't make sense, and I would love it if you could take a minute and be honest with yourself about how you feel. Because it only gets worse when you try to hide or mask it. I've tried it, and it never works!

190

Reflection:
Nobody remembers "easy".

What you're doing in managing T1D is memorable and noteworthy! It takes a lot of hard work. What is one thing that you can learn from today?

_____

_____

_____

_____

_____

_____

_____

_____

_____

_____

_____

_____

_____

_____

TEMPTED TO SKIP INSULIN & LIVE IN DENIAL?

If you're skipping insulin and living in denial, there's a good chance you're dealing with diabulemia. Diabulimia is a life-threatening eating disorder that starts with skipping insulin...and ends in death! If you're struggling with this, it's time to get help.

Kathlin Gordon and Asha Brown at WeAreDiabetes.org can be a great place to start when you're ready to take that leap and start healing this part of your life.

One of their suggestions is to focus on something other than a scale. A scale can be a trigger for a lot of people, and you immediately feel like you're "less than" because of T1D. That leads to trying to take control back, which is where skipping insulin comes in.

Asha says this is where we can start feeling like we're trapped inside of a failed body, and that's where resentment and anxiety can ultimately lead to rebellion. Skipping your insulin is part of that big rebellion.

For us, it may start with "wanting not to have to worry" about diabetes for a while — but skipping your insulin can be very dangerous. In fact, it can destroy your vision, your kidneys, your stomach, and your life.

You're not broken or "less than" — you're frustrated, and I understand. Reach out to the folks at WeAreDiabetes.org and ask for help.

Reflection:
Every day is day one.

The door is shut on yesterday, and you've got a brand new day ahead of you! What is one area that you've grown most in?

_____
_____
_____
_____
_____
_____
_____
_____
_____
_____
_____
_____
_____
_____
_____

WILL MY RELATIONSHIP WITH FOOD CHANGE?

Let's do something together, let's take a little survey about how we feel about food and living with T1D. Give a yes or no answer for each of these questions. You'll add up how many times you've answered yes and figure out how you've done! I'm going to do it, too. There are 10 quick questions.

- Does food stress me out? Yes or no?
- Do I get overwhelmed by food choices?
- Have I ever avoided types of foods completely? Yes or no?
- Does food seem like it has rules to it?
- Have you ever felt guilty for eating something because it would require insulin?
- Has food lost its joy or enjoyment?
- Has food ever felt like a job or math, instead of just eating?
- Does food ever seem like it makes you pay the price for eating it?
- Have you felt left out during gatherings because you think you can't eat something?
- Have you ever skipped a meal because your blood sugars weren't great?

This may help you to realize that living with T1D can change your relationship with food, and it's okay to talk about it!

Reflection:
You're not doing a bad job; you're doing a difficult job.

Numbers are just numbers — not "good or bad." What is something you can celebrate that you did well today?

_____

_____

_____

_____

_____

_____

_____

_____

_____

_____

_____

_____

_____

_____

HOW DO I DEAL WITH ANXIETY & WORRY?

Almost every study I read on the topic of anxiety and T1D points to a fact that I honestly hate. It frustrates me. I don't want it to be true.

If you live with T1D, you have a 20 percent chance of dealing with anxiety versus someone without T1D.

It's all connected. The worry, the fear, being on edge, and managing all the details are how our bodies and minds react to stress. So this book has a bunch of links in the back to resources from professionals whom I trust and respect. They are either living with T1D themselves or have a family member with T1D.

Think about it — how much of your worry or anxious moments are about things happening with your blood sugars vs. what "could happen"? What if you go high, or what if you go low? This is a legit worry every 5 minutes of the day.

The work you do on a daily, minute-by-minute basis is a lot. You're literally trying to stay alive. Who wouldn't develop some degree of anxiety from that?!?!

Reflection:

We are building resilience in us! We're stronger for it and more capable than we ever knew!

Resilience is our superpower, living with T1D. It's building muscles in us that we would never think to work out! What is one thing you can do for yourself today?

_____

_____

_____

_____

_____

_____

_____

_____

_____

_____

_____

_____

_____

_____

_____

SHOULD I BEAT MYSELF UP FOR MY BG LEVELS?

In reality, beating yourself up for not having perfect levels simply doesn't work. It almost always deepens the belief that you're failing. The best thing to do is replace that beating up with empathy.

I've got a ton of empathy for other people's challenges and experiences — but for myself? Rarely. Handling T1D has a little bit to do with how you feel and everything to do with how you behave.

When you see a number or result that just sucks, do this: acknowledge that having T1D may suck; it's uncomfortable, and then choose not to let it get in your way. What if you responded gracefully to the curveballs that T1D throws you?

(Also, remember there are six hormones your body doesn't produce properly! How can you possibly manage a lack of six hormones perfectly? You can't!)

How would you encourage someone else if they told you their blood got out of whack? You'd probably encourage them, right? Tell them there's always tomorrow and they can do it.

Now, turn that around and tell yourself the same thing.

Reflection:

What we celebrate grows.

The things we fist pump and applaud are the things that flourish.
Who has been your biggest support this week?

_____

_____

_____

_____

_____

_____

_____

_____

_____

_____

_____

_____

_____

HOW DO I SET HEALTHY BOUNDARIES WITH OTHER PEOPLE AND MY T1D?

As an adult, I think it's important to set healthy boundaries around living with T1D. People may mean well but have no idea that they are crossing a line with their "advice" and "thoughtful" comments.

Sometimes, it's up to you to educate and teach your friends and family about the basics of T1D. Let's be honest — most people have no idea what insulin does or how your body reacts to food. Teaching them the basics can calm their fears.

Let them know you appreciate their concern; that's genuine, right? I mean, they care about you. Sometimes, they may take it too far, but you need to be honest about where that line is.

Teach them how to help! If my wife Gina knows I'm going low, she knows what snacks to get. She knows where my meter is. And she goes right into that mode. But give people a role in helping us, so they know what to do and not worry as much. It might be as simple as, "You know, Mom, I don't need help with my diet right now. But the thing that would feel most supportive is simply saying, 'I know this is really hard, and I'm really proud of you.'" Give Mom some way to get involved 'cause she loves you!

Reflection:
The highs and lows will happen, but it's what we do with the in-between moments that count!

Away from the anxious moments, the math, the medicine...what did you learn that will benefit you next week and next month?

_____

_____

_____

_____

_____

_____

_____

_____

_____

_____

_____

_____

_____

_____

_____

WHAT IF I'M A CAREGIVER OR PARENT OF A T1D?

When we think about caregiver support, I want us to consider it in a few different categories. A parent of a T1D kiddo. A spouse or partner of someone we love who is living with T1D. A grandparent with a T1D grandchild. A teacher who has a T1D child or young person in their class. And babysitters of young people who have T1D. This is a HUGE group of people who deal with exhaustion, fear and worries, anxiety, and even irritability.

I have links to several things that can help at the back of this book. An ADA Safe at School Campaign to make sure your student has everything they need.

A template letter to teachers and administrators on why your kiddo needs a "low supply box" in their classroom.

A sample Diabetes Medical Management Program that you can fill out with all your kiddo's needs, like doctors' info, medication lists, and what to do if they go low.

And a book by Bonnie O'Neil called, "Chronic Hope: Raising a Child with Chronic Illness with Grace, Courage and Love." I highly recommend it!

Reflection:
Good habits must be established before they can be improved.

You're out there doing the hard work of balancing T1D and life!
What is one thing that's working well for you?

_____

_____

_____

_____

_____

_____

_____

_____

_____

_____

_____

_____

_____

_____

CHAPTER 14

What's next for you?

Scan this before you start reading Chapter 14.

I believe in you. You have the ability to thrive and live with T1D, both. Those things aren't mutually exclusive, and T1D has no right to stop you.

WHAT'S NEXT FOR YOU?

You did it! I knew you had it in you to finish 90 days of learning more about yourself and T1D! Never a doubt in my mind.

What you've read through and journaled about are some of the basics, but definitely not an exhaustive list. You'll likely never get to the bottom of the "learning how to manage our T1D" wishing well. (There is no actual "diabetes wishing well" for the record.) I'd like to welcome you to become a lifelong learner of what makes you tick. Because living with an autoimmune disease like T1D is a whole lot simpler when you keep the mindset that there is so much more to learn.

I want to leave you with some thoughts to help you on your journey. I need this reminder too, so don't think this is aimed at you. I'm writing this down for myself just as much as the person who reads it. The following five things are advice I wish someone had given me a long time ago to help me along the way.

1. Be curious about T1D and your body. Instead of getting frustrated and thinking with finality about highs and lows, food, or activity, ask yourself, "I wonder why that happened?" or "What would happen if I treated this high differently this time?" This isn't just a mindset but a way of living that will pay dividends. Your body and your T1D will change over the years, maybe 50 or 100 different times. You can eat the same thing and get a different response with insulin, and yes, it can be frustrating! But if we ask, "I wonder how this would be different if I just tried _____," then it gets a lot easier because you can't fail as long as you're experimenting!

2. Ask "what now" questions before "why." Many of us go straight to "why" questions when we have a short fuse or when life doesn't go as we thought. And the truth is, we rarely get answers to the "why" questions. If we ask "what now" first, it helps us focus our energy on responding to what happened before we go down a doom spiral of asking why. After we've had a chance to react and take action to remedy whatever high or low we're dealing with, come back to the "why" question with a clear head!

3. T1D doesn't have to be the end of anything. It's the beginning of a lifetime of resilience and determination that makes you stronger. That's not a pep talk; it's the facts. The amount of mental math, concentration, planning and prep that it takes to live with T1D makes you stronger! "More resilient like whoa," says Ginger Vieira. Don't ever let anyone tell you that your life is over or you won't be able to do something because it simply isn't true. I have documented, filmed and interviewed endurance athletes, professional athletes, doctors, lawyers, surgeons and excessively shredded bodybuilders who all live with T1D. Their determination is more substantial than most because they've been handling more challenges than most people ever will. This isn't the end — it's just the beginning!

4. Find community and find it fast! Tell your story to people who will listen and trust a few people by being truly authentic and transparent about the mental and physical side of it. I hid the fact that I had T1D for about 10 years because I was embarrassed, ashamed, and worried about what people would think of me. And then I connected with other people living with the same autoimmune disease I have, and it was like I could immediately hear colors and taste sounds!

I am not joking; my whole world changed because I found my people. The ones who beep, who bleed, who have scars like I do, and who have zero judgment. Finding community should be the #1 thing we do if we're not going to do anything else! It will help tremendously. (There are resources to fantastic groups at the end of the book.)

5. The 42 things that affect diabetes in Chapter 7 is just a guide, and I don't really think that number is entirely accurate. (I have nothing but mad respect for Adam Brown; somebody had to start counting and do what he did!) The list of what affects your blood glucose continues to get bigger, and here is my mentality with it: Look at that list and only focus on the things you can control. That's it! You can't control the weather, humidity, stress on your body, altitude, puberty, allergies or periods! So, skip what you can't control and focus on what you can. Life gets much simpler that way, and it's less to worry about. (I'm looking at you people who complain about the cost of gasoline! Stop it, you're wasting your time and energy!)

I believe in you. I know you can do this. You have the ability to thrive and live with T1D, both. Those things aren't mutually exclusive, and T1D has no right to stop you. I'm running this race right alongside you. I've been there, I'm still here, and I'm not going anywhere. You've got this! Nobody remembers easy! Nobody grows from easy! What you're doing isn't easy, but it's memorable, and you will grow as a person if you let it happen. Now go out there and make some memories by showing T1D who's boss!

(You, you're the boss.)

T1D isn't the main character in your story, you are. It is a footnote or a background character (who likes to mix it up) in your story. You're the hero, and it's been a privilege to be a guide along the way.

CHAPTER 15

Resources that can help!

There are a lot of resources that could help you out. Instead of listing them all out here on paper, where they'll inevitably expire, and you'll get frustrated with me, cut out pictures of Neil from the newspaper and magazines and send him hate mail with nearly illegible handwriting, what do you say we do this?

Here is a giant oversized QR code with a link to an ever-evolving page full of helpful resources that will never expire or go bad, like 2% milk on a hot summer day!

Scan this for resources.

Scan this code. It's like your Golden Ticket to a sugar-free Wonka Chocolate factory of resources without the annoying and imminent gas/diarrhea that sugar-free dreams are made of.

I'm proud of you! This book is only 90 days worth of information, and we both know we'll still need to manage T1D tomorrow. But you're stronger now and more equipped than ever before, and we're in this together.

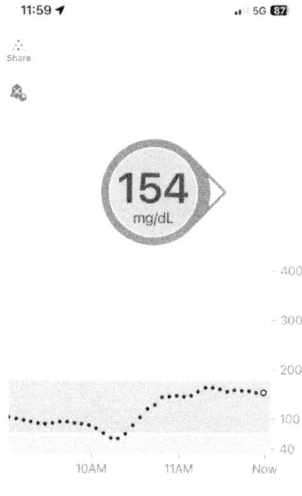

I'm so excited for you that it raised my blood sugar. No lie, this is what my BG was at the time of hitting "publish" on Amazon. I got so fired up thinking about how much stronger you are, and the adrenaline hit me!

In this with you every single day.

Your friend,
Neil C. Greathouse

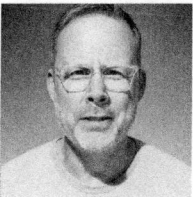

CHAPTER 88

Hidden Chapter

Scan this before you start reading Chapter 88.

This chapter isn't in the Table of Contents or on any treasure map. It's extra. If you want to know what has helped me with my T1D journey more than anything else...this is it. Hint: it's not cinnamon.

"We're either succeeding or learning. Either way, we're growing."

Printed in Great Britain
by Amazon

40273961R00126